SOCIAL ANALYSIS AND THE COVID-19 CRISIS

This book is a collective journal of the COVID-19 pandemic. With first-hand accounts of the pandemic as it unfolded, it explores the social and the political through the lens of the outbreak. Featuring contributors located in India, the United States, Brazil, the United Kingdom, Germany, and Bulgaria, the book presents us with simultaneous multiple histories of our time.

The volume documents the beginning of social distancing and lockdown measures adopted by countries around the word and analyses how these bore upon prevailing social conditions in specific locations. It presents the authors' personal observations in a lucid conversational style as they reflect on themes such as the reorganization of political debates and issues, the experience of the marginalized, theodicy, government policy responses, and shifts into digital space under lockdown, all of these under an overarching narrative of the healthcare and economic crisis facing the world.

A unique and engaging contribution, this book will be useful to students and researchers of sociology, public health, political economy, public policy, and comparative politics. It will also appeal to general readers interested in pandemic literature.

Suman Gupta is Professor of Literature and Cultural History at the Open University, UK. His recent publications include *Digital India and the Poor: Policy, Technology and Society* (2020) and *What Is AI?: A Conversation between an AI Engineer and a Humanities Researcher* (co-authored with Peter H. Tu, 2020).

Richard Allen is Emeritus Professor of English at The Open University, UK. With Harish Trivedi, he wrote and edited *Literature and Nation: Britain and India 1800–1990* (2000), and with Suman Gupta and others, he co-authored *Reconsidering English Studies in Indian Higher Education* (2015).

Maitrayee Basu is Lecturer in Communications and Media at the University of the Arts (UAL), London, UK. Her current research is in the field of digital media cultures, digital identities and political contestations, and digital research methods.

Fabio Akcelrud Durão is Professor of Literary Theory at the State University of Campinas (Unicamp), Brazil. He is the author of *Modernism and Coherence* (2008), *Teoria (literária) americana* (2011), *Fragmentos Reunidos* (2015), and *Metodologia de Pesquisa em Literatura* (2020), among others.

Ayan-Yue Gupta has a BA (Hons) in art history and philosophy from the University of Leeds and an MA in fine art from the Slade UCL and is currently a PhD sociology student at the University of Bristol, UK. He has published a co-authored paper in *Policy Studies*.

Milena Katsarska is Senior Lecturer in American Literature and Culture Studies at the Paisii Hilendarski University of Plovdiv, Bulgaria. Recent publications include the co-authored volume *Usurping Suicide: The Political Resonances of Individual Deaths* (2017).

Sebastian Schuller graduated in comparative literature from Ludwig Maximilian University of Munich, Germany, and currently holds a PhD scholarship of Studienstiftung des deutschen Volkes while working on materialist literary theory in the age of globalization. Schuller has edited an anthology on the rise of the Alt-Right in Germany, *Die Zeit der Monster* (2018).

John Seed taught for many years at the University of Roehampton. His publications on 18th- and 19th-century British social history include *Dissenting Histories: Religious Division and the Politics of Memory in Eighteenth-Century England* (2008) and *The Gordon Riots: Politics, Culture and Insurrection in Late Eighteenth-Century Britain*, co-edited with Ian Haywood (2012). He is also the author of *Marx: A Guide for the Perplexed* (2010).

Peter H. Tu earned his doctorate in 1995 from Oxford University's Engineering Science department. In 1997, he joined the General Electric Research Center, where he is currently GE's chief scientist for artificial intelligence. Tu has 50 issued patents and over 75 peer-reviewed publications.

SOCIAL ANALYSIS AND THE COVID-19 CRISIS

A Collective Journal

Suman Gupta, Richard Allen, Maitrayee Basu, Fabio Akcelrud Durão, Ayan-Yue Gupta, Milena Katsarska, Sebastian Schuller, John Seed, and Peter H. Tu

Routledge
Taylor & Francis Group

LONDON AND NEW YORK

First published 2021
by Routledge
2 Park Square, Milton Park, Abingdon, Oxon OX14 4RN

and by Routledge
52 Vanderbilt Avenue, New York, NY 10017

Routledge is an imprint of the Taylor & Francis Group, an informa business

© 2021 Suman Gupta, Richard Allen, Maitrayee Basu, Fabio Akcelrud
Durão, Ayan-Yue Gupta, Milena Katsarska, Sebastian Schuller, John Seed,
and Peter H. Tu

British Library Cataloguing-in-Publication Data
A catalogue record for this book is available from the British Library

Library of Congress Cataloging-in-Publication Data
Names: Gupta, Suman, 1966– author.
Title: Social analysis and the COVID-19 crisis : a collective journal /
    Suman Gupta [and eight others].
Description: Abingdon, Oxon ; New York, NY : Routledge, 2021. |
    Includes bibliographical references and index.
Identifiers: LCCN 2020028262 (print) | LCCN 2020028263 (ebook)
Subjects: LCSH: COVID-19 (Disease)—Social aspects. |
    Epidemics—Social aspects. | Quarantine—Social aspects.
Classification: LCC RA644.C67 G87 2021 (print) | LCC RA644.C67
    (ebook) | DDC 362.1962/414—dc23
LC record available at https://lccn.loc.gov/2020028262
LC ebook record available at https://lccn.loc.gov/2020028263

ISBN: 978-0-367-63505-3 (hbk)
ISBN: 978-0-367-63661-6 (pbk)
ISBN: 978-1-003-12015-5 (ebk)

Typeset in Bembo
by Apex CoVantage, LLC

CONTENTS

ABOUT THE AUTHORS

Richard Allen is Emeritus Professor of English at The Open University, UK. He was Dean of Arts from 2000 to 2007 and served as an assessor for the UK National Quality Assurance Agency from 2008 to 2016. His career thus combined teaching and research, institutional policy and innovation, management, and quality assurance. His academic interests regularly involve collaboration; with Harish Trivedi, he wrote and edited *Literature and Nation: Britain and India 1800–1990* (2000), and with Suman Gupta and others, he led a research project, the findings published as *Reconsidering English Studies in Indian Higher Education* (2015).

Maitrayee Basu is Lecturer in Communications and Media at the University of the Arts (UAL), London, UK. Her current research is in the field of digital media cultures, digital identities and political contestations, and digital research methods. Before joining UAL, she did her doctoral research on representations of Indian marginalized subjects within new journalistic discourses in India. Her first article, titled 'Representing "The Other India" in Transnational Public Spaces,' is forthcoming in a special issue of the journal *Reserches en Communication*.

Fabio Akcelrud Durão is Professor of Literary Theory at the State University of Campinas (Unicamp), Brazil. He is the author of *Modernism and Coherence* (2008), *Teoria (literária) americana* (2011), *Fragmentos Reunidos* (2015), and *Metodologia de Pesquisa em Literatura* (2020), among others. His research interests include the Frankfurt School, Anglo-American modernism, and Brazilian critical theory.

Ayan-Yue Gupta has a BA (Hons) in art history and philosophy from the University of Leeds, UK and an MA in fine art from the Slade UCL and is currently a PhD sociology student at the University of Bristol, UK. His research: (1) explores ways of improving discourse analysis by drawing upon the philosophy of language and by combining close reading with algorithmic methods taken from natural language processing, and (2) applies the results of this exploration to the area of British government policy making, especially in the Department for Digital, Culture, Media and Sport. He has published a co-authored paper in *Policy Studies*. He is also a practicing artist.

Suman Gupta is Professor of Literature and Cultural History at the Open University, UK. He has led international collaborations across 13 countries and has published 16 monographs, 10 edited volumes, and around 80 scholarly papers. His most recent publications include *Digital India and the Poor: Policy, Technology and Society* (2020) and *What Is AI?: A Conversation between an AI Engineer and a Humanities Researcher* (co-authored with Peter H. Tu, 2020).

Milena Katsarska is Senior Lecturer in American Literature and Culture Studies at the Paisii Hilendarski University of Plovdiv, Bulgaria. Her publications are in culture studies; the politics of cultural translation; the history, sociology and politics of institutional academic spaces; and English and American studies in Bulgaria. Recent publications include the co-authored volume *Usurping Suicide: The Political Resonances of Individual Deaths* (2017). She is presently finalizing a book-length study on the prefatorial discourse surrounding American literature in the socialist context of Bulgaria, *Parapositions: Prefacing American Literature in Bulgarian Translation 1948–1998* (forthcoming).

Sebastian Schuller graduated in comparative literature from Ludwig Maximilian University of Munich, Germany, and currently holds a PhD scholarship of Studienstiftung des deutschen Volkes while working on materialist literary theory in the age of globalization. His fields of research include postcolonial studies, globalization theory, hip-hop studies, Bertolt Brecht, and the aesthetics of Marxism. Schuller has published papers on Brecht and Gisela Elsner ('The Acid of the Materialist Notion of History', *Brecht Yearbook* 43/2018), the relationship of Marxism and literary theory, and German hip-hop, and has edited an anthology on the rise of the Alt-Right in Germany, *Die Zeit der Monster* (2018).

John Seed taught at the University of Roehampton, UK. His research was mostly on 18th- and 19th-century British social history, and publications include *Dissenting Histories: Religious Division and the Politics of Memory in Eighteenth-Century England* (2008) and *The Gordon Riots: Politics, Culture and Insurrection in Late Eighteenth-Century Britain*, co-edited with Ian Haywood (2012). He is also the author of *Marx: A Guide for the Perplexed* (2010). He has been a member of the editorial board of *Social History* since 1982 and was review editor 1982–1994 and associate editor 2010–13.

Peter H. Tu received his bachelor of science degree in 1990 for systems design engineering from the University of Waterloo, Canada. He then earned his doctorate in 1995 from Oxford University's Engineering Science department. In 1997, Tu joined the General Electric Research Center. He is currently GE's chief scientist for artificial intelligence. He has developed various forensic algorithms for the FBI. In addition, he has been the principal investigator for the National Institute of Justice, Department of Homeland Security, and the Defense Advanced Research Program Agency. Tu has 50 issued patents and over 75 peer-reviewed publications.

INTRODUCTION

Having read a first draft of this book, Routledge editors Aakash and Anvitaa declared that it needs an Introduction. This Introduction should address two questions: first, how this book came about, and second, what readers should expect and look for. This is a montage of voices, which might grab readers or throw them off. You need to draw readers in at the beginning, they said. I never quibble with editors, because they are almost always right.

How did this book come about?

In mid-January, Cheng went to Beijing to spend some time with her mother. I had read a couple of reports on this new virus in Wuhan in early January. I mentioned them to Cheng as we waited for her flight in the London Heathrow lobby. She said she had read low-key reports about the contagion on Chinese sites. One doesn't know whether it's as dangerous as SARS. There wasn't much detail. Within a week after she reached Beijing, Wuhan was put into a total lockdown. Beijing streets gradually emptied out; people stopped leaving their apartments; work-unit compounds, offices, and shops were shut; everyone started wearing face masks. International flights from China were being cancelled. In London, I kept a check on the rising numbers of confirmed cases and deaths on a Beijing expat website. Our son rang every now and then to check whether he should be worried.

On 31 January, the farce of Brexit Day took place in London. In my corner of the city, I didn't observe any particular enthusiasm for it. Storm Ciara shrieked through the metropolis soon after. It seemed increasingly uncertain whether Cheng would be able to return on 15 February. The numbers of the infected and dead kept rising in Wuhan but stayed low in Beijing. However, her flight did take off in a gap amidst Storm Dennis and landed in Heathrow a day later. Much of the London

Underground wasn't working, and it rained incessantly as I made my way to the airport to receive Cheng. It felt like a return from a danger zone to relative safety.

Over the next three weeks, the news was about the contamination in China. Racial abuse of persons of Chinese appearance was reported in various parts of Europe, including London. Coronavirus cases started appearing in London; some schools were shut down. A breathtakingly rapid and deadly outbreak in Italy and then Iran gradually took over the front pages of broadsheets. But London remained largely oblivious. I spent most of my days in my study at the university. We went for walks in Richmond Park or along the river, attended concerts, visited our usual cafes and restaurants, met friends. Cheng wondered with a touch of horror what might happen if the virus found its way into India. I was set to visit Delhi on 8 March to spend three weeks catching up on some research and spending time with my parents. Cheng would remain in London. The week before that, I asked at the local clinics and pharmacies whether there were any face masks to be had. The going wisdom at the time in London was that face masks were useless. All smiled and shook their heads a jot ironically when I asked.

On 9 March, I landed in Delhi. There was an undemanding screening exercise to get through, but otherwise not much seemed changed. Over the following weeks, it became evident that London – the United Kingdom – was plummeting into a serious abyss of contagion and deaths, and so was the United States, while the woes of Italy and Iran worsened, and cases started appearing rapidly in other countries of Europe. Delhi now seemed relatively safe, with low numbers of confirmed cases and deaths due to – the media term had changed – Covid-19. Nevertheless, the streets of Delhi began to empty out gradually. Airlines started cancelling flights to and from Delhi, and then a total ban on international travel was declared. My flight was cancelled. I wandered in bookshops, took walks in the hushed local parks, had the occasional meal in strangely quiet restaurants. I ambled into the empty Gallery of Modern Art and spent a couple of hours going through the Gérard Garouste exhibition the day before all museums and tourist sites were shut down. I met friends in empty establishments which one would normally have had to queue to get into. Cheng reported a curious indifference in London as the cases spiralled, and it was becoming evident that the healthcare system was floundering. Our son returned to London from his university in Bristol, which had largely shut down by the 18th. London and Delhi – the United Kingdom and India – formally went into lockdown on the same day, 23 March. I decided to stay in Delhi and see the lockdown out with my parents.

Throughout this period, I was exchanging letters with the friends whose views feature in this book. In fact, these exchanges were parts of ongoing conversations. Some were conversations which had started decades back and showed little sign of fizzling out; others had started a few months earlier and were coming into their own. Each of these conversations had distinct impetuses: shared political and academic interests, the pleasure of having lived together, the familiarity of having worked side by side, curiosity about the different contexts we live in – with as much common ground and difference as friends usually have. It so happened that we were fairly widely dispersed, apart from Delhi (India) and London, also Birmingham (United Kingdom), New York State (United States), São Paulo State (Brazil), Plovdiv (Bulgaria), and Munich (Germany). Each intervention by one of us in the subsequent journal is from one of these locations on a particular date: those are noted at the beginning of the intervention. We were and are all variously engaged in scholarly research but have different kinds of academic backgrounds, mainly in the humanities and social sciences, one in engineering. Unsurprisingly, we share some ideological common ground: all are inclined towards progressive politics; all are non-believers. These details are germane to this book. Every voice is necessarily imbued with its specific tone, experience, identity, proclivities. Our ages range from 27 to 74. Age has a particular part to play in a period when all became sensitized to its significance – vulnerability to Covid-19 appeared graded according to age groups. Other than date and location, however, no other factor bearing upon authorship is marked explicitly for the interventions. It is left to readers to make inferences from their content and tone.

By the middle of March, it seemed to me that the various strands of these conversations, following different patterns and emphases thus far, were beginning to converge. To some degree, this was a thematic convergence. All the concerns and concepts we had been talking about, some of longstanding interest and others more immediate, were becoming conditional to the Covid-19 crisis. It increasingly seemed expedient to ask whether a particular issue or notion was being altered by the Covid-19 crisis, whether it was somehow accentuated, or whether it had in fact become irrelevant. The Covid-19 condition seemingly presented an inescapable grid in terms of which almost any subject or object could be mapped or relocated. Something similar can be traced on a large scale in news media. The diversity of reportage, for different countries, policies, pursuits, conflicts, and productions gradually became reoriented with regard to the Covid-19 crisis. The standard pages on politics, international relations, daily affairs, finance, crime, culture, celebrity, and sports in broadsheets and websites were all talking about the Covid-19 context incessantly and not talking about much else.

This thematic convergence in our exchanges was, however, not moulded by the pervasive media focus. Our dispersed lives and varied interests were not finding connections simply because of a dominant mediascape or by some connecting threads in our academic and ideological inclinations. Utterly extraordinarily, as much in India as in the United States, Brazil, the United Kingdom, Germany, or Bulgaria, the Covid-19 crisis was materially restricting our everyday lives more or less in concert. The process of trying to embed social distancing and impose lockdowns necessarily followed analogous paths. On 11 March, WHO declared Covid-19 a pandemic. As far as the authors of this journal go, social distancing measures and then lockdowns appeared soon after within March. In Bulgaria, a state of emergency was declared on 13 March. New York State, United States, went into lockdown on 16 March; Germany on 22 March; the United Kingdom and India on 23 March; São Paulo State, Brazil, on 24 March. Since we were in conversation with each other, it was also evident to us that we were experiencing this common process in very different, contextually nuanced ways. Just as tabulations of countrywide statistics allow meaningful comparison and, concurrently, differentiation, so the fact that we had the common denominator of lockdown measures served to sharpen the distinctive social dimensions of the cities and towns we were living in.

The experience of being in lockdown wherever we were gave us more time than we would normally have. Even amidst working from home, time often hung heavy. The upheavals that we knew were taking place around and yet beyond our unexpectedly cloistered lives were unsettling. It felt like a time to urgently reassess received ideas and preconceptions, to observe the growing tension in social life all the more keenly. In fact, many of these tensions had been in our conversations for a considerable while and were already at the heart of those ongoing conversations. But now their lines seemed to become taut to the breaking point, some sort of snap seemed imminent. So, as our various conversations converged, our exchanges became lengthier and more searching. The different conversations bled into each other. The observations that were being recorded were of their moment, specific to the day and place they were written in; at the same time, with little nudges and cross-referencing and redistribution, the interventions spoke to each other fluidly and yet coherently and assumed the form of a collective journal. This journal, then, presents a process of thinking – usually troubled, always uncertain – rather than setting out rounded formulations and conclusions. None of us strove to be consistent or sought consensus. Trying to contain the excess of uncertainty and unease made consistency meaningless. Establishing consensus seemed a future task. The journal was simply an attempt to collectively make sense of this extraordinary juncture as it unfolded.

Through this period, lockdowns and social distancing were tracked by a surfeit of messaging, a continuous flow of reiterative announcements, wild rumours, reasonable speculations, and some master narratives. There were two explicit master narratives of crisis through which the Covid-19 restrictions were threaded: a healthcare crisis narrative and an economic crisis narrative. The interventions that form this journal took account of those but were not in their solution-seeking vein. We felt that in these circumstances, critical social analysis is both likely to be in abeyance and to be posed with discouraging challenges; in a modest way, this journal was written to keep our sense of critical social analysis active and alive under unpromising circumstances.

What should readers expect and look for?

As the different conversations converged into this collective journal, some overarching objectives emerged. Generally, the journal was structured through questions being raised and answers being proposed, or, more frequently, methods for reaching towards answers being mooted. Those questions formed steps in the making of the journal. They are stated as they came up in various interventions subsequently. But also, a set of overarching objectives came to inform the journal as a whole, in a more or less continuous fashion. These were:

1   To observe how social distancing and lockdown bear upon prevailing social conditions – accentuating or modifying them – in specific locations;
2   To note whether social distancing and lockdown regimes may portend lasting social changes;
3   To consider what this situation means for various methods and concepts of social analysis;
4   To give a sense of everyday life amidst lockdowns for the locations we live in.

Most interventions were directly addressed to one or two of these objectives, but none were lost from sight throughout the journal. The reader may find the journal veering somewhat precipitously from one location to the other, from the concrete to the abstract, from local knowledge to universal formulations. That's perhaps in the nature of such a juncture, when small matters unexpectedly open into large mysteries and life shoulders death rather more familiarly than we are comfortable with.

Posing questions, as I noted previously, paved the steps which structure this journal. Several kinds of questions come up in the following pages. Some were questions that appeared simply because the situation before us was so unexpected and strange – questions which effectively ask: what is this thing before us? These questions mark the beginning of an enquiry, a search for some way of getting a grip: what sort of contagion is this, why is this different from other contagions, what does it mean to be socially distanced, in what sense is this a crisis or a state of exception? Further, there were questions that followed from that attempt to get a grip. With a bit of a grip, then, these questions tried to strain this juncture through the sieve of familiar concepts – or, alternatively, revise those concepts so that they could penetrate this Covid-19 condition. In this vein: what does it mean to protest in such circumstances, what happens to political practice and policy language, what religious perspective is possible, what is revealed about inequality and poverty, what's happening to our sense of space? At the same time, in yet another vein, questions arose in relation to how the crisis was being dealt with by the powers that be: why this rather than that policy; why is such a measure taken and how will it unfold; who is giving the briefings and directives, with what intentions, what strategies, what fumblings? For us, this line of questioning could not but be troubling, because we have increasingly felt at odds with the high officeholders of our time ('What is an officeholder?' is also a question that's posed). These are the so-called populist leaders of democracies out of joint, with their corrosive regimes and fraught dispensations. President Trump, President Bolsonaro, Prime Minister Modi, Prime Minister Johnson, and their acolytes and cohorts are some of the protagonists of this journal. To us, they seem to suck the Covid-19 crisis into the maelstrom that they are in the eye of, or, perhaps, the Covid-19 crisis seems but a crystallization of the intensifying political crisis which they embody.

But more than these personalities, the rationales which underpin their eminence are of interest. So, questions push towards considering the economic interests and power sleights that endow their antics with calculation – may almost confer sense on their antics. And then there are little questions which float up in the midst of everyday lives. How does this scene I witnessed in the street, this incident in the office or shop, that exchange I had with my neighbour bear upon the overwhelming question of the moment: where is the Covid-19 social condition headed, and where might it end? Does everything have a bearing on this overwhelming question?

These different kinds of questions steer this journal as a collective analytical enterprise – step by step, from one focus to the next. The interventions in this journal are divided into chapters. Each chapter marks a phase when certain questions dominated. The chapters are ordered in a chronological sequence from March to the cusp of May. The chapter headings give a sense of the dominant questions of the phase and period covered: Contagion and Questions, Social Distancing, Lockdown, Suspension of Politics, Of Protests, The Poor and the Way Out, Religion, Exception and Emergency, Real and Digital Space, Tax the Rich. While each chapter heading foregrounds one or two key questions, there is a cumulative drift from one to the next. Earlier responses to questions feed into later responses to other questions. Interventions in different chapters resonate with each other. In particular, questions about the bearing of small everyday observations on the enormity of the global pandemic simmer close to the surface of the journal throughout and occasionally thrust their way to the fore.

Ultimately, this journal presents an attempt simply to think through what we were living through. In retrospect, there are various ways in which this process might appear to be deliberate and designed – a project. This could be considered a deliberative programme of selecting and systematizing from the spontaneous blur of life amidst social upheaval. That would make this journal the product of ideological assertion, wherein we put our feet down firmly on shifting ground, plant an intellectual anchor in the moving sand. Or this could be regarded as a recording project, just archiving what we observed, experienced, and thought over a given period. This would then become a considered contribution to the archive of events – such that future history and imagination can take a singular Event from the archived plethora. Or this may be a project of collective self-management, a coping exercise. We try to control the uncontrollable by wrenching it within theory, pacify the imponderable by pondering, keeping our shared mental equilibrium steady. These are all, however, retrospective ways of thinking about the journal. The truth is, we didn't plan this as a project; we merely plunged into the collective process of thinking and writing as we were plunged into the Covid-19 condition. The journal came together rather than being planned and constructed.

This text is the product – or is it a by-product? – of plunging into analysing what we were living through without allowing for retrospection. At the least, so I think now, with a little bit of retrospection. There is no hindsight as I write this, because the Covid-19 condition continues to evolve; the screw continues to turn. A few days back, shortly after Aakash and Anvitaa asked for this Introduction, a colleague observed in a meeting (online, of course) that he is sceptical of attempts at critical social analysis of the Covid-19 outbreak quite yet. A few years of closure and digesting are needed before well-formulated ideas, meaningful frameworks, and evidenced conclusions can be produced, he said. Don't jump on the bandwagon, you will be in the way, stand by and wait! Give way to the applied scientists and technicians of practical knowledge. The government, the funding bodies, the universities and research institutes, the learned societies are all doing their utmost to engage them. They can and will help solve the extremely challenging problems that are arising. But critical analysis now will only be obtrusively irrelevant. Let the professional problem solvers do their work. At best, critical social analysts should humbly emulate that problem-solving effort, keeping carefully to their place. Perhaps they could be usefully upbeat and encouraging about the consolations of philosophy, cultivate culture for wellbeing, promote art for moral upliftment, undertake to bolster the community spirit . . . I think he was saying that critical analysis could be a problem itself. So, it should be slow, cautious, circumspect, thorough, finished, and meet the approbation of peers and gatekeepers before venturing into the public domain. Otherwise, leave the recording of the present to journalists or propagandists, and leave all the analysing to problem solvers.

For that colleague, this journal will no doubt be an irresponsible text. It does – we do – reject the presumptions this colleague and his ilk make about critical social analysis. This journal is an act of rejection of that view. It is not designed to solve problems but to weigh, dissect, quibble, and indeed to problematize. It is not reportage and does not discover more or less sensational information or putatively offer an objective factual account; rather, it draws upon such reportage in a questioning spirit. It offers no advocacy for or propaganda about any existing political or commercial alignment. It is not an emollient salve to raise the spirits in difficult times. Its modest endeavour is, as I have said already, to keep our sense of critical social analysis active and alive under unpromising circumstances – and to encourage our readers to do so.

Finally, let me give a disclaimer in case of initial misunderstanding. The term 'journal' may lead the reader to anticipate some form of 'life writing', 'testimonial', or 'non-fictional creative writing'. What follows is none of those. We make no claim to narratological art. The following is mainly concerned with concepts and rationales related to a specific social moment. Some of the most imaginative – and imaginary – narratives on epidemics that have influenced me make an allegory of disease. In Albert Camus' *The Plague* (1947), the character Tarrou sees the plague as an allegory for something within the prevailing social order: a systematic dependence on killing. In a larger way, Camus' vision of the plague is of an arbitrary visitation which exposes the essential human condition and the essence of humanity – throws forth an abstract Everyman. In José Saramago's *Blindness* (1997), the epidemic is itself more allegorical than medical, a physical manifestation of social limitations and dysfunction. In what follows, there's no place for allegory. Covid-19 is a biological fact which is at the crux of a global social phenomenon. Nothing more.

Suman Gupta
15 May 2020

1

CONTAGION AND QUESTIONS

Summary: *As a springboard for discussion, attention is drawn to the prevalence of TB as the most deadly infectious disease of our time. A parallel for TB to the measures for Covid-19 contagion is imagined. This offers an opportunity for interventions to dwell upon the distinctiveness of the Covid-19 outbreak, consider the different attitudes to TB and Covid-19, or reflect upon responses to the latter in specific locations and national contexts. Views from specific contexts are variously revealing of concerns foregrounded therein and of what the authors felt was significant on their own account. Later in the chapter, a number of questions are posed by way of structuring this journal's approach to the crisis. Some immediate reactions are given, which effectively point toward themes which appear in subsequent chapters.*

Suman Gupta (16 March 2020, Delhi, India)

Tuberculosis is the deadliest infectious disease of our time. The WHO estimates that in 2017 around 1.6 million persons died of TB and in 2018 1.5 million; each year around 10 million people are infected.[1]

Suppose all the governments of the world decide that today is Day 1 for tracking the spread and fatalities of TB. They give out three numbers on Day 1: this many were confirmed as infected by TB today, this many died, and this many recovered. Each day thereafter, they keep adding up the tally of the day to the total to that point from Day 1. Or maybe this is done every hour. These three cumulative numbers keep growing for one week, then two weeks, then two months, and onwards. These numbers are blasted out on every TV channel, news outlet, office notice, government report, subway poster, bulletin board, social network feed . . . in a continuous shrill drone. Soon after Day 1 is declared, every country in the world sets up police and military and medical detective forces to track the pathway of

TB contagion for every case reported; anyone suspected of possibly being in contact with someone who might have TB is quarantined; gigantic TB-suspect treatment centres are set up; symptom-screening is routinized in airports; docks, borders, and TB-intensive countries are blocked off . . .

TB has been around for a while. It's a matter of putting a Day 1 and reeling out three numbers with no context.

Let's get perverse. Let's appoint a Day 1 for counting cumulatively the number of affected people and fatalities for any potential cause of death and keep bombarding everyone with these two figures – for domestic violence, traffic accidents, police custody deaths. . . . If one puts one's mind to it, any of those might some time assume the proportions of a dangerous epidemic.

The trick, of course, is that we think we can prudently avoid the police or the abusive partner or speeding vehicle, but we can't be sure that we can avoid TB. The initial symptoms are of the sort that everyone has experienced possibly once a year or more – sore throat, coughing, sneezing, low fever, muscle aches – not far from a severe case of hay fever. It is unassuming enough initially to be very close, very possible, almost inside you already. Its very familiarity now suddenly makes everything and everyone suspect; every situation opens up vulnerabilities. Ritualizing preventive measures – wash your hands, cover your mouth, and so on – assume a kind of magical efficacy without guarantees – it's a bit like salvation: it's good to do it, but doing it doesn't mean you will be saved. Inanimate things assume a threatening spirit. Anything with a surface (and what's a thing without a surface?) suddenly comes alive with bacteria that might kill me, anywhere, in public transport, film halls, school classrooms, shops, protest meetings, offices. A philosophy of 'social distancing' develops, avoidance of strangers and foreigners first and then avoidance of friends and comrades. Studied isolation and atomized communication become not just de rigueur but necessary.

Peter H. Tu (17 March 2020, Niskayuna, New York State, United States)

I take your point that TB is a bad actor. A few years back, my brother stopped by my house for a friendly visit just after returning from a Doctors Without Borders stint in Africa. It turns out that he contracted both malaria and tuberculosis. We all had to get tested for TB, and my brother had to go on a regimen of medication and evaluation. Of course, the upside is that TB is usually treatable if one has access to the right drugs. Unless there is significant close-quarters interaction, it is not too transmissive. In general, the older a virus or bacterium gets, the less lethal it becomes. So let me push back ever so slightly on your hint of 'We are blowing this thing way out of proportion' . . .

The problems with Covid-19 are:

1   It is too new, and so we have no real remedy other than ventilators for those who are really suffering – in general, the flu and TB are treatable.
2   Unlike the flu, which has a mortality rate of 0.1, Covid-19 may have a mortality rate of up to 2% (this number is not really known).[2]

3   Each person that catches Covid-19 infects on average two other people (this is high), hence the doubling or exponential nature of this disease.[3]
4   Of those that catch it, 15% may require hospitalization – if they don't get access to a hospital bed with a ventilator, mortality rates go up really fast. This is why China had to build multiple hospitals in a matter of a week.[4] In the United States, there are roughly 1 million hospital beds, of which 75% are currently in use.[5] In the United States, healthcare is a business. They follow the argument that you don't build a church for Easter Sunday. So the current fear is that the exponential growth of infection + 15% hospitalization rate could easily overwhelm the nation's capacity for intensive care. Hence the desire to flatten and spread out the curve.
5   Of course, Covid-19 comes from the heart of the orient and thus has the taint of being intrinsically evil, if not existential in its menace.

We just got an email that one of the kids in the local elementary school has just tested positive for Covid-19. All children, parents, and staff have now been asked to go into a 14-day quarantine.

I have always been a fan of the zombie film genre. I particularly enjoy the *Walking Dead* franchise. One can't help but feel that there is something zombiesque going on here. In particular, children and teenagers are more frightening than ever. Since they seem to be more resilient to this affliction, they take on an air of carefree-super-spreaders. Being over 50 and having a mild case of asthma, I find myself counted amongst those that must cower in the shadows in mortal fear of such inadvertent monsters. It is like being trapped in an endless Halloween. One blessing is that J and his posse very much enjoy the online gaming lifestyle. Other than the fact that his soccer club has had to end its season prematurely, I don't think he even notices that we are in a lockdown situation. Maybe evolution has elected to select for the gamers . . .

K is in her element. Once she got wind of this virus (December or January timeframe?), she has been in preparation mode. While I would not put us in the ranks of panicky hoarders, we do have an impressive collection of canned foods and dried goods. She decided to upgrade our refrigerator and has purchased a large standalone freezer unit. On my part, I have now transformed the living room into a remote office of sorts. I have two card tables, a power bar, my laptop, and a spare screen. I am just a few clicks away from commandeering the house printer.

It's only day 2 of my voluntary cloistering, but clearly I too am beginning to get bored with this arrangement . . .

John Seed (18 March 2020, London, United Kingdom)

You are absolutely right, Suman. I suppose it's the difference between a long-term situation and a sudden EVENT. It's the sudden explosion of Covid-19 that blew health provision in Northern Italy apart.[6]

And it matters in a different way as an event because Covid-19 is democratic. Suddenly the rich and powerful are as at risk (more or less) as the poor and powerless. Money no longer functions as part of their immune system. This was a lesson the British bourgeoisie learned in the 19th century. Starvation wages and filthy slums had a direct effect on them in the form of cholera, typhus, and so on.[7] They and their families were not safe even in green well-policed suburbs on the edge of town. Public health and medical facilities for all were grudgingly and slowly conceded.

So will the US bourgeoisie finally learn it now? I doubt it. In the United Kingdom, there's panic-buying of toilet paper;[8] in the United States, apparently there's been panic-buying of guns.[9] I gather there are still those who think it's fake news. The right and need to carry arms and the hostility to a national health service express the same bone-headed individualism. I suppose if they could invade foreign countries individually they wouldn't need to pay taxes for an army. But war and pillage require a degree of social cooperation and collective action.

It's interesting to see how fear and stupidity combine to generate amazing paranoid fantasies and delusions. I saw a YouTube video about the pandemic being a strategy for planned depopulation.[10] And another of a scary American 'news' presenter claiming it was part of a conspiracy to harvest organs by the Chinese government.[11] Plenty of people think it's a Chinese biological weapon, and plenty of others think it's a US biological weapon planted in Wuhan. It's nice for them that they think some branch of humanity is in charge.[12]

I read a message from a nurse in a big Liverpool hospital this morning saying that all leave has been cancelled, patients are being discharged, all non-urgent provision is cancelled, and the hospital is being put on a war footing. So it looks like the bomb of exponential growth is about to explode in the United Kingdom. It presumably goes off in London first.

My self-isolation is interrupted today for an emergency visit to the dentist. I almost look forward to it. I could get stir-crazy by the middle of next week

Milena Katsarska (18 March 2020, Plovdiv, Bulgaria)

The military, headed by General Ventsislav Mutafchiyski, and the Chief Prosecutor Ivan Geshev here are doing a good job of dealing with the Covid-19 threat firmly.[13] Their major problem is tackling the two extreme positions of unthinking bravado and irrational panic. I quite appreciate how they arrested (1) a small group of drivers returning from Austria who broke the quarantine rule and went to have drinks in a local pub[14] and (2) some British student from the Plovdiv Medical Academy who was spreading fake news online about a school with 200 cases he allegedly heard about at a briefing.[15] Similarly, with regard to panic, they are holding constant information bulletins to repeat *ad nauseam* that neither copious amounts of toilet paper nor kilos of food packages nor heaps of antibiotics are necessary because there's a regular supply. The Bulgarian people are unlikely to be left starving. Bulgaria doesn't have a population of unemployed or homeless millions, really. There's also a serious clamp down on hoarding, as reports have trickled in on the exorbitant prices being charged for disinfectant, masks, and so on. Bulgaria is small and easily manageable (or should be), and the fear is really that collectively 'we' are prone to behaving like Italians or Spaniards and might tip the balance in the directions they did.[16]

R became visibly calmer yesterday after the operational HQ announced that due payments for small businesses will be postponed and the government will meet 60% of their salary costs in the next three to six months. This is okay, given that the rule of thumb is that employers – with the blessing of employees – usually declare up to 60% of the real salaries they give/receive. That will naturally raise the question of where that budget gap will be compensated from. An easy guess is: from precisely the areas that got closed down immediately – state-sponsored culture and education. I will be on high alert as to how these tweaks will play out in the long run and be on the lookout as to what exactly is happening in a 'state of emergency' for which, incidentally, Bulgaria has no real legal framework, outlining the dos and don'ts.[17]

I will check how far we got in terms of securing the payment for this month for our part-time university teachers. They are in a vulnerable position, as their income depends on the shitty contracts that mean no-classes-no-money. However, since we made moves to go into a sort of online teaching mode, they should be able to keep that. This miniscule instance shows how important it is that everyone, I mean every single person, has a guaranteed base salary, which is not too difficult to accomplish within, again, such a tiny country.

But the speed with which the whole rhetoric went in the direction of 'taking care of one's own' – be that nationally, family-wise, or of the same class background – is worrying. What is happening with refugees in camps or outside them and among other such vulnerable groups? To take another example: since Bulgaria has impeccable broadband connection, school education went online quickly. That alerted people to the fact that there are areas 'with compact populations' (read: ghetto-like structures) where the access is not the same. There are families in which existing devices cannot really cover every single member simply because all adults and children have to be using them simultaneously. The brave new world of technology – hooray! Let's study and work online from home is neither so shiny an idea and nor so unproblematic. However, in recent history, we have had political turmoil disrupting education on a large scale, that is, the student occupation and general strikes in the 1990s that lasted for over a month.[18] These were compensated without much havoc in times of a total lack of technological facilities. Although the coronavirus is heat resistant, the moment the weather gets warmer, the seasonal flu will disappear (that's currently exacerbating the mess), and it will be easier to manage.

In any case, I think in Bulgaria, if there were elections tomorrow, they would elect General Mutafchiyski – the General – immediately for whatever post he would like for himself. A post could even be invented for him. Bulgarians are such suckers for a 'strong hand'; if it's military, all the better. He has even eclipsed Prime Minister Borisov to a great extent, not to mention that President Rumen Radev must be feeling quite isolated. That's probably why he is meeting with the trade unions today. The game here is played in the name of the 1.358 billion Euros that each country can have as aid from the EU emergency fund.[19] If that's a capped entitlement, it is very problematic because Bulgaria cannot really be compared to much larger countries or countries that are having decisively harder times these days. But this pan–European fiscal solidarity opens unprecedented opportunities for financial speculation.

P.S. Later I did have a closer look into the 60% government promise for salary compensation, and it is in fact just for show and quite suspect.[20] That is for layoffs due to business stagnation. As matters currently stand (without any emergency situation or funds), there is anyway a mechanism of 80%–100% compensation in case of layoffs for which the social security funds should have money anyway. So what exactly is the government 'promising' so generously?

Richard Allen (19 March 2020, Birmingham, United Kingdom)

Thanks for your meditation on TB. It sent me off to the WHO website, which was quite chastening, notwithstanding it didn't contain the number of deaths from police assaults or the number caught up in proxy wars.

It's difficult then to get the Covid-19 crisis into perspective, both because it's happening NOW and because it's still quite new. On the long-term positive side, it seems to be akin to things for which vaccines have been successfully developed, and on the short-term negative side, there doesn't seem much that can be done about it now. Except, of course, have good hospital care and – though it's somehow not polite to say this very loudly – the NHS seems to be doing not particularly well by comparison with the German system.[21] All the strategy of recent years of somehow magically pushing treatment into the community and actually reducing the number of beds available is coming back to haunt us, and one hopes the planners too. We are in a different situation from China, but there are moments of thinking with envy about the state delivering food to citizens as one queues for rapidly dwindling supplies in supermarkets. We older folk can be forgiven for thinking we are also expendable; support the young and the workers – and no doubt the bankers who are selling stocks themselves or sitting by their computer-driven systems.

We are not entirely on enforced sequestration and can go to the shops and take exercise. I'm taking my isolating area into my car and thence to my allotment where I can easily be socially distanced in the middle of the plot. The threat of boredom does hang heavy, however. Our book group has suspended itself in the middle of reading *Northanger Abbey* for the next meeting so we're wondering how we can exchange views remotely. Once that is done, I've the last volume of the Elena Ferrante quartet to read. The digital TV channels are so far keeping us supplied too with afternoon 'classics' or just old cinema enabling the revisiting of the culture of the 1950s when I was a child and certainly didn't go to the cinema.

John Seed (19 March 2020, London, United Kingdom)

The figures for Covid-19 cases are entirely useless. Hardly anybody is being tested in the United Kingdom unless one arrives at a medical facility as a suspected case. They are guessing that there may be as many as 50,000 cases by now in the

United Kingdom. But nobody has a clue. It is thus impossible to make comparisons between two random samples of two populations. The high figure of cases for Germany (and low death rate) is probably because of a more systematic testing regime rather than their better health facilities. Their demography is not significantly different either.

I think figures for deaths are probably a more useful index of the spread of the virus. But even then, it is very much a rough guess. Some poor old sod with lung cancer gets Covid-19 and his exit is accelerated. But how is his cause of death consistently evaluated between different physicians and coroners? And anyway, for purposes of comparison, it needs to be correlated with the size of the population. In a few weeks, deaths in India will probably be a tidal wave.

The apparent arrest of Covid-19 in China may be a temporary respite. They can't live in lockdown permanently. As soon as social interaction multiplies, it will begin to spread again. Back to square one. The virus is now endemic to the human population, and everybody will get it at some time in the next few years. It can't be eradicated. Vaccination might blunt its impact in the long term. I would probably be better off getting the damn thing now – though we don't know if it has long-term health implications. There is talk of permanent scarring of the lungs. There's also talk that younger people who smoke are more vulnerable to complications.

It's a gigantic disaster, and we will be paying for it in reduced living standards for a very long time. I see Spain has nationalized all its private hospitals.[22] I wonder what kind of compensation will be paid – over-generous, I expect.

My diary is empty now for weeks ahead. Feels very odd. They are expecting an upsurge in pregnancies and divorces.

Sebastian Schuller (19 March 2020, Munich, Germany)

I find what you write about TB intriguing, but I do not totally agree with it.

My experience is this. People have become nervous in the way you described. I myself have become very cautious, and both K and I (we are living together, since the lockdown may start at any moment) have this need for constant self-reflection, much as you describe it. This is like a religious ritual. Every cough makes you think, every touch is a transgression, and every contact with the outside is a brush with an evil world. One feels a need, communicated via different media and through politics, to restrain oneself, to follow the rites and keep oneself away from the world like an 11th-century hermit.

So, in brief, there's a religious air around all that as you described it.

But I experience the opposite as well. Not only are people openly defiant – we see people celebrating in the park all night long now, pretty much like the orgies during the Black Death[23] – I also experience a new sense of communality and collectivity.

Take the solidarity committees I am involved in. There are now 1,500 people registered in an organization, led by communists, that did not exist one week ago. Every quarter has several committees; people are helping wherever possible.

On a personal level, I think people are far more interested in one another. In the few days of prescribed isolation, I had more deep conversations with my friends than in years. Not only about politics; we talked about personal stuff, never mentioned before, perhaps because we all share this sense of danger. This may sound perverse and is probably a very white and first-worldly view, but I think that for many of my generation, this is the first time that we have experienced a major disturbance. This is a moment of history, which might very well mean the end of neoliberalism as we know it. The market development is going that way, I feel. So, that's why this creates anxiety, though we all realize that for people in the global south, this may be a more common experience, the imminent possibility of many deaths. But the current situation may also result in the rise of a collective consciousness of history.

Suman Gupta (20 March 2020, Delhi, India)

I am still in Delhi, wondering how and when I'll get back. The government here has just banned all international flights, incoming and outgoing.

Apart from using TB to give a hypothetical parallel to the coronavirus reaction, there's a more direct side to the comparison.

TB has recently caused an average of 1.6 million confirmed deaths each year; it used to be higher around the year 2000. Around 10 million people are estimated to become infected each year – I suspect many infections and deaths are not reported.[24] There's a vaccine, and it can be treated with antibiotics. This has been carrying on for many years; the annual mortality rates used to be higher, and *still* the number of deaths hovers around 1.5 million.

So far, in three months, Covid-19 has caused around 10,000 deaths (Italy and China account for over 7,000 of those). 245,000 people have been infected in three months.[25] The mortality rate is around 4% (maybe higher in Italy, Iran, Spain, and the United Kingdom). There's no vaccine or treatment yet.

What you have to ask yourself is: how come, with a vaccine and treatment, TB continues to have those extraordinary figures? And you have the answer: because it largely happens in poor regions among poor people. People haven't bothered to try and really stop it.

The key point about coronavirus is that it has predominantly affected rich countries – China, North America, the EU. The cost/loss that has gone into it already is astronomical. And not just by the key affected rich countries. In India, around 450,000 persons die of TB every year, I read recently in a news report.[26] So far there have been four deaths from Covid-19 in India. India has already spent infinitely more resources on the latter than it has ever spent on TB.

Watching the Indian coronavirus response is an interesting pastime. The chief minister of Delhi yesterday banned all gatherings of 50 or more, except for weddings.[27] For weddings, it is okay for 100s to congregate. Why? Because these are happy people? Because weddings are immune to the spread of coronavirus?

Apparently there are devout Hindus dotted around the country, drinking the piss of holy cows to ward off the virus.[28]

There's a strong moral bent in India's response to the thing. The relatively low figures compared to EU, United States, China – rich countries like that – is something to foreground. They cause anxiety, but they also make Indians feel good compared to those Western snobs. The government is making serious efforts, and that's why the figures are low, is the inference to make.

Peter H. Tu (20 March 2020, Niskayuna, New York State, United States)

As opposed to Indian righteousness, I find myself shocked at American incompetence. . . . These days, I am comforted by the process of making lists. So here is a set of administrative outrages in bullet form:

- Two years into his administration, Trump fires the White House pandemic response group (put together after the Ebola crisis).[29] He suspects that they were harboring deep-state Obama sympathies.
- Trump sees the whole Covid-19 situation through the lens of how it affects him personally – he declares it to be a Liberal Hoax that is over-hyped and meant to injure his re-election prospects.[30] Fake news!
    - ○ Fox News starts pushing the idea that this is overblown liberal conspiracy.[31]
    - ○ Trump loyalists start making fun of Covid-19; at the Conservative Political Action Group (CPAC), Republican Congressman Matt Gaetz mockingly dons a gas mask. It turns out that both he and another Republican congressman, Louie Gohmert, become exposed to Covid-19. Matt goes into a 14-day voluntary quarantine.[32] Louie refuses to self-quarantine and returns to Congress.[33]
    - ○ On Sunday, Republican congressman from California Devin Nunes tells everyone that they should continue to go to restaurants though the governor Gavin Newsom ordered a shutdown.[34]
    - ○ The governor of Oklahoma, Kevin Stitt, tweeted a picture of his family in a crowded restaurant.[35]
    - ○ Young Republicans flock to bars and beaches during spring break to show their support for Trump and defiance against education and expertise.
- The WHO offers Covid-19 testing kits to the United States. Trump refuses the offer, since his people view international assistance as a form of weakness.[36] With no testing, the United States shifts from the South Korea model to an Italian experience.
- Trump starts to fret about a stock market crash. Unfortunately, he had already given away a huge tax cut to corporations, which they used for stock buyback and CEO compensation. Having blown a hole in the debt and forced the Fed to lower interest rates to almost zero (all to juice the economy for

his re-election),[37] Trump finds himself with little to no ammunition for the economic fallout to come.

- States cry that there is a critical shortage of ventilators, beds, and protective equipment. Trump snarls that the federal government is not a sourcing service.
- Starting to realize the gravity of the situation, Trump reaches into his old bag of tricks and starts to refer to Covid-19 as 'the Chinese Virus'. White House minions use the nickname KungFuFlu.[38] Trump suggests that China should pay for damage done to the US economy. He also uses the crisis to increase fear about the US/Mexican border – let the hate crimes roll.
- The army corps of engineers essentially put a stop to the Ebola epidemic by building field hospitals in Africa. Right now, they are sitting in the barracks while US hospitals are quickly being overrun.
- Ninety-five percent of Republicans say that Trump is doing a fine job handling this crisis. Trump gives himself a grade of 10 out of 10.

There is an argument that until we come up with some sort of vaccine, we may face recurring waves of infection. The nearest example of this was the Black Plague, which lasted for centuries. During one of these waves, Newton had to flee Cambridge and hide out in his country home. It was during this period of isolation that he came up with optics and calculus.

NY State (hardest hit of all states) has gone to a 100% shelter-in-place position. All non-essential businesses must work from home. Luckily, I can do this type of thing. But if the whole laboratory shuts down . . .

Peter H. Tu (21 March 2020, Niskayuna, New York State, United States)

Here in New York State, all non-essential work must be done at home. Yesterday a person at my office was diagnosed with Covid-19. He was returning from a business trip abroad and was self-quarantining before returning to the office. So, as far as we know nobody else at the office was affected.

To be fair, I suppose I am honor bound to put caveats to my previous list of iniquities, and also to be fair to add to it:

- While Trump did disband the national security epidemic response team, he was not the only one to do so. The history is something like the following:[39]
  - Clinton started the epidemic response team
  - Bush Jr fired them
  - After 9-11 and the anthrax scare, Bush Jr reinstated the team
  - When Obama took office, he fired them
  - After the Ebola crisis, Obama reinstated the team
  - When Trump took over, he fired them
  - So I guess from a we vs. them situation, this one is kind of a wash . . .

- The most recent outrage: after getting a classified briefing in early February about how bad Covid-19 was going to be, two Republican senators, Richard Burr and Kelly Loeffler, went on television touting the Trump line that everything is under control and that there is nothing to worry about. Meanwhile, they are both feverishly selling off their stocks and warning their fat-cat friends to do the same.[40] The ethics committee will soon start an investigation into insider trading. One of the senators is the wife of the man that runs the New York Stock Exchange.

For the last three years Trump has gotten away with just reacting based on his short-term desires and appetites. Jared Kushner has told him that this was just like the flu, and so all he did was shut the border. While not particularly progressive, shutting the border probably bought some time. It's a shame that we did practically nothing with it. It seems that if the President does not want to hear bad news, nobody is willing to lift a finger. . . . I am not sure if one can expect anything more from two sons of wealthy real-estate developers, one slightly more fraudulent than the other.

Suman Gupta (21 March 2020, Delhi, India)

Questions I am contemplating:

- What is the relationship between the financial crisis, the refugee crisis, and the coronavirus crisis?
- Can profits be made from the coronavirus contagion? Who might make them?
- Does the pandemic have any bearing on nationalism and fascism? Can it be read as a vindication of impregnable borders and no migration?
- Can 'social distancing' become an ideological principle?
- What is the political economy of statistics in the coronavirus context? That is, what do the statistical indicators highlighted in the media indicate to whom?
- What does the pandemic mean for the university? (A matter of both public and self-interest for me.)

On the last, it has turned almost all universities into e-learning centres for a while, and I suspect to some degree permanently. There are some businesses which see a good opportunity in this large scale move to online in universities. These are higher education online-teaching platform providers (for massive open online courses or MOOCs) – like Coursera, EdX.[41] They have been serving universities offering online courses already by giving a platform and templates for online course delivery for, of course, some returns. They have done something clever now. They have made some of their offerings free to help out universities affected by the virus situation. This has been hailed as an extraordinary act of generosity. That's the freebie that will get the clients in – they may be set to make a killing.

John Seed (21 March 2020, London, United Kingdom)

Trump never ceases to amaze me . . .

Your first question is the big one, Suman – unanswerable, except, perhaps, as a way of synthesizing the others into an unstable conjuncture.

Profits can be made from Covid-19. The supermarkets are having a great time; sales are up on a range of items; pharmaceuticals are booming. I suppose the manufacturer or copyright owner of the new vaccine will make a fortune (another fortune). The press and media in general (talking-head physicians in particular) must be profiting. Against this, the losses of a broad range of services will be catastrophic – restaurants, theatres, cinemas, gyms, city-centre clothing stores, professional sports clubs, and so on. I expect a lot of these companies will never come back. A whole bourgeois way of life may disappear. No more gyms or middle-range restaurants. The urban landscape is going to look very different by the middle of 2021. And our massively reduced incomes are not going to provide enough demand for replacements. Goodbye Pizza Express and cheap Italian lunches in Kingston.

Social distancing: apparently the Queen is going to practice social distance now. So we are informed. No more buses or chip shops or nights in the local pub for her majesty. Social distance was always an ideological principle, part of the management of relations between classes. First-, second-, and third-class railways carriages, for instance. The boxes in theatres. And, more broadly, social segregation in the modern city. All of these had roots in fear of contagion. British cities were swept by epidemics of typhus, cholera, and all kinds of dangerous diseases. This was a key force behind suburban development. So this will push us back to stricter social segregation – though, of course, disguised as simply the effect of the market. The Savoy is free to all.

And this will also have geopolitical forms, as another of your questions suggests. The phasing of the pandemic may well mean that Europe and the United States are beginning to recover by the end of 2020 just as parts of Africa and Asia are heading into their climacteric. Borders will be tightly maintained. I can't see the EU preventing an upsurge in internal borders. And the extra-European will be identified as a particular threat. Again there are lots of precedents for this in the 19th century. I wonder if there's going to be particular anger directed towards China and the Chinese. It's going to produce a fruitful soil for all kinds of racisms, nationalisms, and fascisms.

So, yes, Covid-19, the refugee crisis, the disintegration of the EU, revitalized right-wing nationalisms, and a new huge economic depression are going to be articulated together in all kinds of horrible ways. The 2020s are not going to be a good time anywhere.

Ayan-Yue Gupta (21 March 2020, London, United Kingdom)

The financial crisis is the trigger of austerity, which made faith in 'optimization' as efficiency into habitual common sense. So, public services like the NHS were 'optimized', meaning they use minimal resources during 'normal' service and are completely unable to deal with anything beyond 'normality'. There've been worsening winter crises in the NHS every year, and now the NHS will struggle to deal with coronavirus. I don't know about the links to the refugee crisis.

Yes, I think fascists will definitely try and take advantage of this. Already happening with the conspiracy theories about the virus being manufactured as a bioweapon by China. The left are also trying to take advantage of this, hopefully they will succeed. Leftwing news channels are using the epidemic to argue against dogma of 'optimization' and in favour of more resources for public services, basic income, and so on. I have seen quite a few mutual aid groups spring up, so the Kropotkinites[42] are about, too.

An ideological principle as in an unquestioned faith in the goodness of social distancing regardless of context? I'm not sure how social distancing could come to be thought of as good outside an epidemic. People like to socialize too much for this.

At the moment, just from my own bubble of information, the statistical indicators highlighted show the disease spreading quickly. The numbers of hospital beds and ventilators are being cited to show how the government is unprepared. That narrative might change, though. Are you trying to figure out whose interests the published figures serve?

Do you think numbers of non-virtual students will be permanently reduced after the pandemic?

Richard Allen (21 March 2020, Birmingham, United Kingdom)

These are apt questions; some immediate thoughts follow. Other questions might be added to them. Can governments keep control of the common sense in the agenda? What happens if numbers of medical professionals start to die because they don't have enough safety equipment?

Can profits be made from the coronavirus contagion? Who might make them? I'm sure profits are already being made through algorithmic trading on the stock exchange.[43] More directly, the company making the first vaccine should make some money. Beyond that, I wonder. A comparison with the results of the Ebola outbreak might be instructive. Can more money be made from a pandemic that hits developed countries as opposed to under-developed?

Does the pandemic have any bearing on nationalism and fascism? Can it be read as a vindication of impregnable borders and no migration? I'm sure the answer to the second question is 'yes'. And you might add 'racism' as involved in nationalism and fascism. Trump is already repeatedly calling it the 'Chinese virus'.[44] Can one seriously expect Matteo Salvini[45] not to make anti-immigrant capital out of the outbreak that has hit his own heartland so hard?

Can 'social distancing' become an ideological principle? Interesting. It seems more likely to remain a part of the Policy Makers' rational arguments. How can I be socially distanced in queuing for the supermarket or a bus? It might be thought to be a North European thing, but even then, I wonder.

What is the political economy of statistics in the coronavirus context? That is, what do the statistical indicators highlighted in the media indicate to whom? The statistics in the media largely reflect the Policy Makers' agenda. At the moment, they seem to capture the number of deaths and the number of cases, but since in the United Kingdom testing is woefully limited, the details exist without a context – rather like the number of people killed/injured in a road crash or affected by flooding. It's a truism that coronavirus kills people who were going to die anyway, but the loose references to people who have died having 'underlying conditions' doesn't help.

Milena Katsarska (22 March 2020, Plovdiv, Bulgaria)

There will be a lot of work unpicking and tracing current moves in an analytical mode once the dust settles.

As of yesterday morning – which I gathered only at 8pm during the BNT evening news – movement between big cities is being heavily monitored. There are controls at every exit/entrance and a total ban on lingering in parks. Meanwhile, a private laboratory has started testing (nobody reported on what they charged) and sending results directly to the test subjects without consulting the 'steering committee'. That had pissed off the General big time.

How can one structure a response path to your first question about the relationship between the three crises?

1   At one level, they all share the designation 'crisis', which marks an extraordinary/exceptional juncture against 'everydayness' or 'normality'. In this respect, one may tap into the respective contexts of normality (what was economic normality, migration normality, disease/mortality normality) prior to the tipping point at which a situation is designated as a 'crisis'. What is the relationship between such a designation and objective reality?

2   At another level, these follow one after another with sort of five-year gaps. Viewing them as a succession of crises, highlighting their sequence (out of all other smaller crises or points of tension, testing boundaries of some sort), already designates that particular array of three with specific weight. I suppose you had reasons for not putting Brexit there? Is that because it is subordinate to the first two or a fallout from them, or because it is a regional, not a global, issue?

3   Nevertheless, if we adopt the succession of those three without circumspection or with some qualifications, then we have established certain relations of a temporal sequencing and a narrative with three scenes/episodes. As such, we might have: (1) a unifying principle that it is the underlying economy that's central (yeah, political economy, but emphasis on financial/economic principles); (2) a rhetorical link in substance and as shaped through media or government discourses between them, one after another.

Should we explore point 3 or all three? Even if it's just the latter, one can go in the direction of one trope and see how it fares across them all. Take, for instance, the expression of government (centralized power, the remit of government, executive action/inaction, control, freedom, etc.) and see whether there are commonalities and differences (or rather continuities and rifts) between the manifestations of government power at all three junctions. Or one could take a different order of a concept – choose between 'threat', 'security', 'border', 'movement/mobility' (let's not take 'freedom' because that will be uselessly abstract, I think) – and see how the way in which those feature and change at each juncture of the three crises is indicative of certain relations.

The bottom line might well be that it will be safe to move capital (and goods) across borders, but the new profit-oriented bright future will leave movement of bodies only as the controlled privilege of an elite. In that process, two problems might be solved: of overpopulation and of an ageing population – worldwide and especially in the 'western world'. The ageing population here might not be viewed particularly as a burden of the social side of the economy (although there's that, too) but as one that might be useless or harder 'to convert' to an entirely virtual economic world, hence unproductive in the new order.

Notes

1 For the 2018 WHO figures, see www.who.int/news-room/fact-sheets/detail/tuberculosis; for the 2017 figures www.who.int/gho/tb/epidemic/cases_deaths/en/ (accessed 28 May 2020).

2 See Rachael Rettner, 'How does the new coronavirus compare with the flu?' *Live Science*, 13 May 2020, www.livescience.com/new-coronavirus-compare-with-flu.html (accessed 28 May 2020).

3 Chris Canipe, 'Covid-19's exponential growth', *Reuters Graphics*, 17 March 2020, https://graphics.reuters.com/HEALTH-CORONAVIRUS-GROWTH/0100B5KL438/ (accessed 28 May 2020).

4 Jessica Wang, Ellie Zhu and Taylor Umlauf, 'How China built two coronavirus hospitals in just over a week', *Wall Street Journal*, 6 February 2020, www.wsj.com/articles/how-china-can-build-a-coronavirus-hospital-in-10-days-11580397751 (accessed 28 May 2020).

5 Jayme Fraser and Matt Wynn, 'US hospitals will run out of beds if coronavirus cases spike', *USA Today*, 13 March 2020, www.usatoday.com/in-depth/news/investigations/2020/03/13/us-hospitals-overwhlemed-coronavirus-cases-result-in-too-few-beds/5002942002/ (accessed 28 May 2020).

6 Miles Johnson and Davide Ghiglione, 'Coronavirus "tsunami" pushes Italy's hospitals to breaking point', *Financial Times*, 11 March 2020, www.ft.com/content/34f25036-62f4-11ea-a6cd-df28cc3c6a68; Michelle Bertelli, 'Coronavirus pandemic piles pressure on Italy's health system', *AlJazeera*, 18 March 2020, www.aljazeera.com/indepth/features/coronavirus-pandemic-piles-pressure-italy-health-system-200317171603485.html (accessed 28 May 2020).

7 Mary Wilson Carpenter, *Health, Medicine, and Society in Victorian England* (Santa Barbara CA: Praeger, 2010); Pamela K. Gilbert, *Mapping the Victorian Social Body* (Albany: State University of New York Press, 2004).

8 Andy J. Yap, 'Coronavirus: Why people are panic buying loo roll and how to stop it', *The Conversation*, 6 March 2020, https://theconversation.com/coronavirus-why-people-are-panic-buying-loo-roll-and-how-to-stop-it-133115 (accessed 28 May 2020).

9 Ed Pilkington, 'US sales of guns and ammunition soar amid coronavirus panic buying', *Guardian*, 16 March 2020, www.theguardian.com/world/2020/mar/16/us-sales-guns-ammunition-soar-amid-coronavirus-panic-buying (accessed 28 May 2020).

10 'Coronavirus: Depopulation agenda', 1 March 2020, www.youtube.com/watch?v=8d7acZSB_sY (accessed 28 May 2020).

11 'Coronavirus reveals China's darkest secret', *China Uncensored*, 14 March 2020, www.youtube.com/watch?v=0ZgYqrZoXCs (accessed 28 May 2020).

12 'Is coronavirus a secret Chinese bio-warfare weapon? fact check', *India Today*, 17 February 2020, www.youtube.com/watch?v=-hD-PWN5UN0 (accessed 28 May 2020).

13 In Bulgaria, the effort to combat the pandemic was fronted by Ventsislav Mutafchiyksi, a professor of the Military Medical Academy and major general of the Military Medical Academy, who was appointed as head of the National Operational Headquarter to Fight the Coronavirus Pandemic. He and his team, with Public Prosecutor Ivan Geshev, appointed as such in late 2019, were responsible for determining the strategy and delivering daily public briefings. This was unlike the other contexts this journal covers, where political heads of state and governors/ministers seemed at the forefront of efforts and undertook the public messaging. The heads of state in Bulgaria played a relatively subdued role in this instance. That includes President Rumen Radev, who had assumed the position in 2018 as an independent candidate supported by the Bulgarian Socialist Party, and Prime Minister Boyko Borisov of the centre-right GERB party, in his third term then, having first assumed the position in 2009. Radev also has a military career and is a major general; Borisov had the rank of general as chief secretary of the Ministry of Interior 2001–2005 before founding the GERB Party.

14 'Четирима шофьори са арестувани за нарушаване на карантината', *Rubric Politics, Healthcare,* Клуб *Z,* 14 March 2020, https://clubz.bg/95615-chetirima_shofori_sa_arestuvani_za_narushavane_na_karantinata (accessed 28 May 2020).

15 'Foreign medical student in Bulgaria's Plovdiv held after spreading fake Covid-19 claim', *Sofia Globe,* 16 March 2020, https://sofiaglobe.com/2020/03/16/foreign-medical-student-in-bulgarias-plovdiv-held-after-spreading-fake-covid-19-claim/ (accessed 28 May 2020).

16 'Coronavirus: Europe now epicentre of the pandemic, says WHO', *BBC*, 13 March 2020, www.bbc.com/news/world-europe-51876784 (accessed 28 May 2020). An informally held idea of the time was that Southern European countries tend to be culturally accustomed to more person-to-person contact than the Northern, which might explain their greater vulnerability to the virus.

17 For a discussion of the legal framework which appeared after this was written, see: Radosveta Vassileva, 'Bulgaria: COVID-19 as an excuse to solidify autocracy?' *Verfassungsblog: On Matters Constitutional*, 10 April 2020, https://verfassungsblog.de/bulgaria-covid-19-as-an-excuse-to-solidify-autocracy/ (accessed 28 May 2020).

18 This refers to what is regarded as the 'first democratic student protests' and university occupations of 1990 (throughout the summer at a national level), leading to the resignation of Prime Minister Petar Mladenov (after being recorded on camera saying 'let's call the tanks'), and the student protests of 1997 that lasted 30 days in January and contributed to the toppling of the government of Prime Minister Zhan Videnov. For context, see: Iveta Todorova-Pirgova, 'Symbols and images of "Evil" in student protests in Sofia, 1997', *Cultural Analysis*, 2, 2001, 107–28; Tom Junes, *Students Take Bulgaria's Protests to the Next Level. Can They Break the Political Stalemate?* (Vienna: Institut für die Wissenschaften vom Menschen, 2013), www.iwm.at/transit-online/students-take-bulgarias-protests-to-the-next-level-why-the-student-protests-could-break-the-political-stalemate/#_ftn29 (accessed 29 May 2020).

19 Krasen Nikolov, 'България получава 1.35 млрд. евро от ЕС за борба с коронавируса', *Euractiv,* 15 March 2020, https://euractiv.bg/section/%D0%BF%D0%BE%D0%BB%D0%B8%D1%82%D0%B8%D0%BA%D0%B0/news/%D0%B1%D1%8A%D0%BB%D0%B3%D0%B0%D1%80%D0%B8%D1%8F-%D0%BF%D0%BE%D0%BB%

D1%83%D1%87%D0%B0%D0%B2%D0%B0-1-35-%D0%BC%D0%BB%D1%80-%D0%B5%D0%B2%D1%80%D0%BE-%D0%BE%D1%82-%D0%B5%D1%81-%D0%B7%D0%B0-%D0%B1%D0%BE/ (accessed 29 May 2020).

20 For a clarification on this which appeared after the intervention was written, see: Kalina Krastanova, 'Bulgarian government adopts wage subsidies to support business during crisis', *CMS Law-Now*, 2 April 2020, www.cms-lawnow.com/ealerts/2020/04/bulgarian-government-adopts-wage-subsidies-to-support-business-during-crisis (accessed 28 May 2020).

21 There were a few articles expressing concern about the state of British health services compared to other countries, including Germany, at the time: James Melville, 'Welfare cuts have left UK undefended against coronavirus', *AlJazeera*, 13 March 2020, www.aljazeera.com/indepth/opinion/welfare-cuts-left-uk-undefended-coronavirus-200312193147678.html. More straightforward comparisons appeared somewhat later, for instance: Chris Morris, 'Coronavirus: What can the UK learn from Germany on testing?' *BBC*, 11 April 2020, www.bbc.com/news/health-52234061 (accessed 28 May 2020).

22 Adam Payne, 'Spain has nationalised all of its private hospitals as the country goes into coronavirus lockdown', *Business Insider*, 16 March 2020, www.businessinsider.in/politics/news/spain-has-nationalised-all-of-its-private-hospitals-as-the-country-goes-into-coronavirus-lockdown/articleshow/74658200.cms.

23 See David Herlihy, *Black Death and the Transformation of the West* (Cambridge, MA: Harvard University Press, 1997), p. 64.

24 For the 2018 WHO figures, see www.who.int/news-room/fact-sheets/detail/tuberculosis; for the 2017 figures and other statistics www.who.int/gho/tb/epidemic/cases_deaths/en/ (accessed 28 May 2020).

25 These are the figures given on 20 March 2020 at *Worldometers*, www.worldometers.info/coronavirus/#countries.

26 'These diseases kill many more than coronavirus', *Times of India*, 17 March 2020, https://timesofindia.indiatimes.com/india/these-diseases-kill-many-more-than-coronavirus/articleshow/74670863.cms (accessed 28 May 2020).

27 'Coronavirus scare: Weddings okayed, but Delhi CM Arvind Kejriwal urges people to think twice', *Times of India*, 17 March 2020, https://timesofindia.indiatimes.com/city/delhi/coronavirus-scare-weddings-okayed-but-delhi-cm-arvind-kejriwal-urges-people-to-think-twice/articleshow/74664688.cms (accessed 28 May 2020).

28 PTI, 'Coronavirus: Group hosts "cow urine party", says COVID-19 due to meat-eaters', *Hindu*, 14 March 2020, www.thehindu.com/news/national/coronavirus-group-hosts-cow-urine-party-says-covid-19-due-to-meat-eaters/article31070516.ece (accessed 28 May 2020).

29 Lena H. Sun, 'Top White House official in charge of pandemic response exits abruptly', *Washington Post*, 11 May 2018, www.washingtonpost.com/news/to-your-health/wp/2018/05/10/top-white-house-official-in-charge-of-pandemic-response-exits-abruptly/ (accessed 28 May 2020).

30 Nancy Cook and Matthew Choi, 'Trump rallies his base to treat coronavirus as a "hoax"', *Politico*, 28 February 2020, www.politico.com/news/2020/02/28/trump-south-carolina-rally-coronavirus-118269 (accessed 28 May 2020).

31 Inae Oh, 'Fox news can't decide if coronavirus is a real threat or an impeachment scam', *Mother Jones*, 10 March 2020, www.motherjones.com/media/2020/03/fox-news-coronavirus-impeachment/ (accessed 28 May 2020).

32 'Coronavirus: Quarantined congressman flew with Trump on Air Force One', *Guardian*, 9 March 2020, www.theguardian.com/us-news/2020/mar/09/matt-gaetz-coronavirus-cpac-quarantine (accessed 28 May 2020).

33 Justine Coleman, 'Gohmert returns to congress despite possible coronavirus exposure after physician recommendation', *The Hill*, 9 March 2020, https://thehill.com/homenews/house/486703-gohmert-returns-to-congress-despite-possible-coronavirus-exposure-after (accessed 28 May 2020).

34 Katie Shepherd, 'Public health experts say stay in. Devin Nunes and other defiant officials say, "It's a great time to just go out",' *Washington Post*, 16 March 2020, www.washingtonpost.com/nation/2020/03/16/coronavirus-nunes-bars/ (accessed 29 May 2020).

35 Paul LeBlanc, 'Oklahoma governor who faced backlash over "packed" restaurant tweet now declares emergency', *CNN*, 16 March 2020, https://edition.cnn.com/2020/03/15/politics/oklahoma-governor-deleted-tweet-coronavirus/index.html (accessed 29 May 2020).

36 Arman Azad, 'WHO and CDC never discussed providing international test kits to the US, global health agency says', *CNN*, 18 March 2020, https://edition.cnn.com/2020/03/18/health/who-coronavirus-tests-cdc/index.html (accessed 29 May 2020).

37 Howard Gold, 'A feckless Fed, huge deficits and poisonous politics have brought us to a crisis', *Marketwatch*, 16 March 2020, www.marketwatch.com/story/a-feckless-fed-huge-deficits-and-poisonous-politics-bring-us-to-a-crisis-2020-03-16 (accessed 29 May 2020).

38 Barnini Chakraborty, 'Trump doubles down on "China virus", demands to know who in White house used phrase "Kung Flu".' *Fox News*, 18 March 2020, www.foxnews.com/politics/trump-coronavirus-china-virus-white-house-kung-flu (accessed 29 May 2020).

39 For details, see: Ken Dilanian, Dan De Luce and Andrew W. Lehren, 'From Clinton to Trump, 20 years of boom and mostly bust in prepping for pandemics', *NBC News*, 13 April 2020, www.nbcnews.com/politics/national-security/clinton-trump-20-years-boom-mostly-bust-prepping-pandemics-n1182291; Dan Diamond, 'Inside America's 2-decade failure to prepare for coronavirus', *Politico*, 11 April 2020, www.politico.com/news/magazine/2020/04/11/america-two-decade-failure-prepare-coronavirus-179574 (accessed 29 May 2020).

40 Kadhim Shubber, 'Two US senators sold shares after receiving virus briefing', *Financial Times*, 19 March 2020, www.ft.com/content/e3a82b44-6a3f-11ea-800d-da70cff6e4d3 (accessed 29 May 2020).

41 Rhea Kelly, 'Coursera, EdX offer free access to courses for universities impacted by coronavirus', *Campus Technology*, 12 March 2020, https://campustechnology.com/articles/2020/03/12/coursera-edx-offer-free-access-to-courses-for-universities-impacted-by-coronavirus.aspx (accessed 29 May 2020).

42 Followers of the anarchist-communist philosopher Pyotr Kropotkin (1842–1921).

43 Using a computer programme with a set of instructions to place a trade in stock exchanges without human intervention.

44 See note 38.

45 Leader of the Italian rightwing anti-immigrant party Lega Nord, who had served as deputy prime minister of Italy and minister of the interior between June 2018 and September 2019.

2
SOCIAL DISTANCING

Summary: *Some of the conceptual nuances of social distancing as a response to the pandemic are raised. In particular, the distinction between active and preventive treatment is noted, the part played by modelling is outlined, potential social transformations are considered, and the older sociological sense of the phrase is recalled. A discussion on the reliability of statistics follows. Other implications of social distancing are also picked up thereafter, in terms of language usage, political interests, and demographic features. An attempt to classify the principal kinds of political responses to Covid-19 is made at the end of the chapter.*

Suman Gupta (23 March 2020, Delhi, India)

1   There's no vaccine or cure for Covid-19. So, there are two forms of treatment. There's *preventive treatment* for those who are yet unaffected: enabling enhanced sanitary practices, social distancing, and quarantining the infected. There's *active treatment* for those who are infected: the management of symptoms and the hopeful administration of medicines usually used for infections which show similar symptoms.

2   If we consider the reported numbers of the infected who have recovered or died from Covid-19, we can get a sense of the importance of active treatment – that is, after infection. The figure for confirmed cases is so dependent on chance and scale of testing that it doesn't provide a sufficient basis for saying much. But death and recovery seem to be reasonably indicative, at least of an official record. Where death figures per X of the population are relatively high and recovery figures per X of the population are relatively low, we may infer that active treatment is inadequate. At the least, they indicate closure of a

record of death and cause of death, or closure of the record of a condition and its cessation.

China's effectiveness in engaging the virus has tended to be put down to strongly centralized implementation of *preventive treatment* in the international media. That doesn't explain the high incidence of recovery, which is due to *active treatment* – China invested most heavily in opening new hospitals and arranging medical care for an immensely increased number of patients. The United States and United Kingdom at present have atypically high numbers of deaths and low numbers of recoveries. This is probably evidence of indifferent attention to active treatment – or the greatest inability or lack of will to provide active treatment. However, these might be variables that change with time: it might well be that after three months, UK and USA death and recovery figures will be proportionally similar to China's now.

3 If the *active treatment* is muted, all that's left to push vociferously is the *preventive treatment*. From the governmental point of view, the two directions of treatment have different thrusts. Active treatment has to be led by medical experts; preventive treatment is largely an act of state, and political leaders take centre stage. Active treatment involves planned infrastructural investment; preventive treatment principally calls for compensatory spending. Active treatment is easier if strong investments have already taken place and infrastructure exists; preventive treatment here is the path that appears after the fact. In the United Kingdom – and in India, where I am at present – the media is currently totally focused on preventive treatment, and there is very little reported on active treatment. The main phrases that have surfaced by way of preventive treatment are 'social distancing' and 'self-isolation'. The latter is for those who may reasonably suspect that they could be infected; the former is the general preventive measure (along with enhanced sanitation habits). Let me focus on *social distancing*.

4 Social distancing involves enforcing reduction of direct contact between persons to a minimum within a community (however that's defined as a spatial collective) and also restricting movement across communities (from moderated porosity of borders to cordon sanitaire). The effectiveness of this for influenza pandemics is much studied. The usual way of gauging effectiveness is to model pandemic situations within a typical or representative community and across representative communities. The model can then be used to track normal contact patterns across different levels of membership which can correlate to a normal pattern of infectious spread (exponential for Covid-19). Then targeted adjustments towards minimizing those normal contact patterns can be modelled to obtain measures for consequent reduction of infectious spread – and therefore of morbidity and mortality. Social distancing as the central governmental strategy for influenza pandemics was adopted, it seems, around 2004–2006. In this period, a good example of the kind of modelling that recommends social distancing is found in R. Glass et al., 2006 ('Targeted Social Distancing Designs

for Pandemic Influenza').[1] In 2006, too, US Homeland Security released its *National Strategy for Pandemic Influenza*, which put considerable weight on social distancing. This divided up preventive treatment into two categories: transmission interventions (face masks, hand hygiene, etc.) and contact interventions (the area of social distancing) – for the latter, measures such as:

> substituting teleconferences for face-to-face meetings, the use of other social distancing techniques, and the implementation of liberal leave policies for persons with sick family members, all of which eliminate or reduce the likelihood of contact with infected individuals. Interventions will have different costs and benefits, and be more or less appropriate or feasible, in different settings and for different individuals.[2]

Both models and strategies for social distancing have been honed since, especially with regard to resource and expertise allocations and organization – but the general principles hold.

5   Social relations between government and polity seem to take an interesting turn when social distancing is the principal and focalized response to a pandemic. (1) On the one hand, the government becomes licensed – a state of exception – to act in ways which would be otherwise regarded as ham-handedly authoritarian. At the same time, the polity – of which each uninfected member now feels (or could be persuaded to feel) vulnerable – demands authoritarian measures, and implements/regulates/polices those measures of their own initiative to some extent. (2) On the other hand, the failures of the government's record – past and present – tend to become magnified. Along with current compliance, a general sense of dissatisfaction may set in. The government is likely to ratchet up its authoritarian benevolence accordingly. (3) On the one hand, the government assumes an extraordinary responsibility. On the other hand, it seems that responsibility for failures ultimately have to do with the nature of the polity – its disobedience, its weaker elements (the elderly, children, anti-social components, etc.).

6   At the present juncture, social distancing opens up two particular potentials, which we could think of as collateral but possibly long-term effects. First: in 2006, teleconferencing instead of face-to-face meetings seemed the limit of compensatory recourse to technology of US Homeland Security; in 2019, an entire sphere of parallel online sociality exists alongside day-to-day physical sociality. Social distancing becomes a matter, to a great extent, of transferring as much of physical sociality to online sociality as possible. In this respect, social distancing seems to fall in synch with a wider move already underway. Ever greater proportions of work and social interactions have been moved online as a matter of policy: meetings, classrooms, conferences, transactions, reporting, contracting, archiving, record keeping, and so on. The reasons for this have been economic: the more that work, in particular, can be shifted online, the less expensive it is for employers – saves costs of space, insurances, management

of physical persons, transport costs, and so on and increases opportunities for downsizing and casualization. However, work is still largely set to an idea of collective presence and endeavour. Social distancing as preventive treatment in an emergency could become a bridge to comprehensive and maximal online working as a habitual productive practice. For employers, such a move also has further benefits. The online space is a totally recorded and monitored space (no more whispers in the corridors) and therefore more closely manageable. Social distancing as an emergency measure would naturally be relaxed gradually and perhaps finally only to the extent that a leap forward in online work and productivity becomes set and quickly normalized.

7   Second: Over the last decade, by degrees, conservative nationalist authoritarian – tendentiously far right – governments have been emerging through democratic procedures around the world. Some of the common ground these share are neoliberal economic arrangements, active preferment of moneyed elites, conceptions of homogeneous ethnic and racial nations, hostility to gender equality, hostility to minorities, hostility to evidenced critical reasoning, religious worldviews, militarism, closed borders, and strong anti-immigration and xenophobic rhetoric. The pandemic and social distancing as preventive treatment could be turned into metaphors for those convictions by such governments – and such alignments generally. The pandemic and social distancing measures may bolster the populist push which underpins the recent success of rightwing alignments.

8   At a broader and more abstract level, it is perhaps worth recalling that social distancing is not a concept which originates in medical and healthcare circles – it is grounded in the social sciences. It is a mode of conceptualizing spatiality in social relations generally: between different strata of society, between intellectuals/elites and lower classes/workers, between variously alienated or integrated individuals and communities, within institutional hierarchies, and so on. The broad principles were laid out usefully in Karl Mannheim's *Essays on the Sociology of Culture* (1956), especially Part III, The Democratization of Culture. This puts a perspective on social distancing in terms, on the one hand, of a concept of normal social proximity and, on the other hand, of a notion of 'existential distance' (that which an individual feels towards another irrespective of social conditions). Mannheim's main thesis in this regard was that in pre-democratic society, social distance was a perspective and practice exercised by elites/intellectuals towards lower orders or others – an insertion of what he called 'vertical distance'. According to Mannheim: 'Democratization means essentially a reduction of vertical distance, a de-distanciation'.[3] It seems ironic that the potentials marked in 6 and 7 could insert social distancing as a norm of democratic society once its preventive-treatment recourse becomes redundant or is made, at some level, permanent. That won't be a de-distancing but perhaps a maximization of horizontal distance between persons.

John Seed (23 March 2020, London, United Kingdom)

Well, let me offer a few questions and qualifications.

Regarding point 2: there is no way of making meaningful comparisons between cases, deaths, recoveries between different nation-states. Germany is testing far, far more than anybody else. And I have my doubts about how they are evaluating cause of death. It may well be the case that German healthcare is better than the British or other parts of Europe. And it may be that the Chinese have been very effective in both prevention and recovery. But I don't think anything other than very cautious conclusions can be drawn from such erratic data.

Anyway, what do we know about the pre-existing health of the respective populations? My guess is that smoking and diabetes (and pre-diabetes) are more prevalent in Southern Europe. The latter (but probably not the former) are also probably more prevalent in the United Kingdom and United States than in Germany – or China, South Korea, and Japan. Italy and Spain probably have an older population too? So, pre-existing populations surely have different vulnerabilities to different kinds of infections? It may be that a longer-term effect of this pandemic will be to put further pressure on companies to reduce sugar and carbohydrates in the Western diet. A cheap unhealthy mass-produced diet is now rocking the very foundations of the global economy. Covid-19 is not, it seems, an especially virulent infection – it simply exposes the vulnerability of an ill-fed and overweight population.

I am not throwing a bucket of icy scepticism about all the available data. On the contrary. But it seems to me that you jump too fast to a conclusion. The uncertainty of the evidence warrants no more than cautious suggestion and speculation.

Incidentally, I really don't see how lockdown can work in the long term. It's a temporary measure to manage the pressure on healthcare facilities. As soon as China and South Korea and other states relax constraints on social interaction, it's going to flare up again. Some kind of 'herd immunity' argument may actually be right in the long run. The hubris of states – perhaps especially the Chinese and US states – may not like this exposure of their impotence.

I have no qualms about your other points, which begin to lay out sophisticated arguments about some of the political implications of social distancing. I don't buy the Mannheim argument, though. Social distancing was not undermined by democratization – something which isn't really occurring to the late 19th century anyway. That's the whole burden of Marx's critique of the state/civil society distinction.[4] Men are equal in the transcendent sphere of the state, one man, one vote. But the secular sphere of civil society is riven by every kind of material, economic, and social inequality. Class was and is still materialized in social distancing: housing and urban social zoning has a huge literature. Social distancing has always been integral to class society. Individuals are trained from a young age to detect the nuances of class in voice and visual cues and respond appropriately. And space has always been managed to preserve social distinctions. The 19th-century bourgeoisie were obsessed with the fear of contagion and infection and with ensuring that a safe distance was preserved between them and the polluted masses. Our cities are living embodiments of that insecurity: disease, riot, collective insanity blur into each other. The hot breath of the mob!

Suman Gupta (23 March 2020, Delhi, India)

On Mannheim, I totally agree: vertical distances have never been especially diminished by formal democracy. Seemed too good an opportunity not to exploit the irony, though.

On statistics: as a rule, people argue hardest about the figures they don't like and go along with the figures that suit their preconceived notions; also as a rule, there's almost nothing that is really robust statistics in the social sphere: if one were looking for hypothetical flaws (as you are here) you can always find them. Give me any set of social statistics and I can point out how shaky it probably was in elicitation, tabulation, analysis. So, an inference from social statistics, despite its scientific appearance, is generally little more than a plausible indication, perhaps a provocation to act in one way or another. Unlike statistics in the natural sphere (scientific), a trend in social statistics is extremely difficult to repeatedly confirm.

But the death and recovery figures have a legalistic validity that the total number of confirmed cases do not. Causes of death and diagnoses of causes from which recovery take place are legally fixed for hospital records and death certification.

Milena Katsarska (23 March 2020, Plovdiv, Bulgaria)

What are the terms/phrases other than 'social distancing' that overlap and slip within the domain of usage? 'Social isolation' seems to gesture towards psychological effects due to the social environment (work from home, online shopping, old age/disability preventing access, etc.). 'Interpersonal distance(s)' nods towards intercultural communication, with an eye on trends in dominant cultural group (of the middle class, the dominant ethnicity, the national character). What else?

Taken on its own, though, 'social distancing' now is a call to actively do so. The onus of responsibility is within the domain of individual ability and action; that is, each person must decide whether 'to remove herself from society' so as to (1) preserve herself and (2) reduce the possibility of harming others. There's more to that, though, it seems to me. It might superficially connote a reduction of this phrase to bodies in a spatial relation to each other, but 'social' is deployed there instead of 'self' (as in 'self distancing') – that implies something while obscuring that implication at the same time. And I am not even mentioning that a call for social distancing the way it is imperatively made now and repeated like a mantra nevertheless is an impossibility for some social groups and beyond their control. Say, where a family of eight has one large room and one toilet to share, or one's work is effectively on a factory floor or in open floor plan offices, or one lives in a shared facility, such as a dorm. How much exactly does this imperative call for 'social distancing' depend upon me?

Fabio Akcelrud Durão (25 March 2020, São Carlos, São Paulo State, Brazil)

Suman, you are pointing to transformations that may be momentously terrible, a deepening in the social dynamics of domination. This is certainly true, of course. I would only call your attention to three factors:

1   Active treatment will come in due course, and it will be a huge source of profit for the pharmaceutical industry. The problem with epidemics is that active treatment necessarily lags behind the outbreak of the disease. And another flu-like illness will most likely emerge in the near future, possibly more lethal than Covid-19. So social distancing is in a certain measure unavoidable.
2   The changes in everyday life are so drastic and have such strong economic impact that, as you say, a considerable social instability ensues. Such instability can have unpredictable political results. Here in Brazil, it is amusing to see the big media starting to use the first-person plural, something I haven't seen since the military dictatorship. They are starting to become afraid of the populace. The effect of the coronavirus on densely populated favelas and the reaction of the residents there is already causing great anxiety.[5] The government is considering decreeing a state of siege but will probably not do it, because it could generate even more unrest. It may be that the left leaves this crisis strengthened. Or it may not . . .
3   Social isolation may indeed lead to heightened labour exploitation, but slavery-like levels of daily work are already being demanded of Uber drivers and food deliverers (Uber and Ifood are the biggest employers in the country).

President Jair Bolsonaro went on national TV to follow in Trump's footsteps. Their advisors and strategists must be the same. He basically urged people to go back to work and fill the streets, for schools to resume classes, and so on, so that the economy won't stop.[6] The state governors are going in the opposite direction, as is Congress and the Supreme Court. The next few days will get to the boiling point. Bolsonaro is probably trying to stage a coup.[7] He might be waiting for signs of unrest to make his move, which will come either through people starving or the accumulation of corpses dying from the virus. It's amazing how off the radar he is from any understandable policy of organizing the economy and taking care of the virus at the same time. Bolsonaro can only think of both as mutually exclusive areas. Interestingly, Bolsonaro is also on a collision course with mainstream media, either TV Globo[8] or he will fall before 2022. As I always say, one can't complain of boredom in Brazil – no *Weltschmerz* around here.

Maitrayee Basu (25 March 2020, London, United Kingdom)

The division of the management of Covid-19 responses between active and passive treatments is very useful and clearly demarcates the medical and expert-based responses and sociopolitical responses. In terms of disciplinary focus, this provides a very good framework to focus one's analysis. One clarification that might be needed is regarding population demographics. As more data emerges about the population affected, including cures and deaths, it might be useful to factor in age and general health based on geographical regions as well into the argument. Because at the moment, I have seen it being argued that the reason for Italy's high death toll is a huge elderly population and their proximity to younger people who act as carriers of the virus.

Suman, you then focus on social distancing from points 3 onwards, which is understandable, as that is the focus of media and political discourse as well as, and also consequently, of a majority of organizational and public discourse (based on online traces – emails, social media posts and discussions, reported conversations). This is also the focus of a lot of paranoid and neoliberal stress management affective discourses – which has been my own focus during this time. I am also interested in the sharing of motivational and sentimental posts, as well as angry ones, that project a seemingly generalizable shared experience, thus expressing a desire for some sort of sociality – political or otherwise. Whereas these discourses draw from the official and heavily reported ones on mainstream news media, they cannot be conflated. Moreover, the pace of emergency measures being introduced necessitates a frenzied sharing of information on various communication channels by individuals who see themselves as necessary nodes of a post-broadcast era distributed-communication landscape. There is an affective response of shutting down and being overwhelmed, which Akwugo Emejulu and Leah Bassel (2020) connect to the politics of exhaustion: 'To declare exhaustion . . . is to hail the equally exhausted to build solidarity'.[9]

I think you are spot on when it comes to surveillance and the emergency switch to online spaces – I have been thinking of the number of people who are using Amazon now, as well as online grocery services. There is also a new app from researchers at King's College which asks UK citizens to give data towards a public-led mapping of Covid-19, and people are in these circumstances happy to do this. This diverges from the use of such apps in South Korea, as it relies on voluntary trade-off of data for public security with potentially more ethical use of the data during and after the emergency. However, there is also a potential for more mature conversations about data in public space, and collective use of data, compared to what we have seen in alarmist predictions about data in recent years (which probably set the stage for people to be more aware of ownership and rights to data in the first place, which is good).

Similarly, work cultures being shifted online does present the possibility of a shrinking of collective awareness that social relations at the workplace presents. Being part of the University and College Union strike action just before the Covid-19 lockdown in the United Kingdom, as well as actively involving myself in the various socializing opportunities it presented – picketing, running our branch Twitter Comms, leafletting and talking to staff and students, teach-outs, starting a WhatsApp group for striking department members, lunches and rallies – has given me a good opportunity to reflect on these various spaces of collective organization. At UAL, we suffered from not having a physical union space or even a student union space, which universities like Goldsmiths and SOAS have and which would have made it possible perhaps to organize more coherently and for longer lengths of time. Whilst switching to online teaching in the last few weeks of term (for us there are still eight weeks left after Easter break!) we are asked to present a step-by-step plan of action for each module, which must be approved by managers and presumably could be checked more easily given the recorded nature of all teaching activities to enable more discipline and surveillance; as you say, this was already happening to a great extent.

Having read some digital ethnographers recently, as well as sociologists working on the internet using qualitative methods, the conflation of online spaces as a 'place' only seems to be too simple; rather, it is a place only sometimes. The complexity of cultural activities taking place on the Internet may not map as comfortably on to global and local, so there is scope to see how the modes of surveillance and governance map onto this terrain in terms of not just scale, as in reach, but also evenness.

But my first thoughts on points 7 and 8 in your notes are: whereas the distancing of sociality that the government-enforced sanctions imply an immediate withdrawal from one's physical surroundings and neighbourhoods (those that you signify as horizontally linked), the rhetoric also emphasizes a heightened duty of care and responsibility, and therefore a different type of awareness, for other inhabitants in these spaces. I am interested to see how this awareness is sustained or transformed as the crisis deepens, as seems inevitable in the United Kingdom and United States and most likely in India. I am also wondering how the new discourse on 'key workers' highlighting the porosity of geographical and social stratification in cities would change the greater political discourse. There's a lot of the marketing around such spaces focused on aspects that made certain bodies and agencies invisible – for example, daily wage domestic workers in gated communities. The awareness of viral infections linking different localities perhaps also brings to the front the inequalities but also the interlinkedness of these spaces.

Sebastian Schuller (25 March 2020, Munich, Germany)

The last days were strange here in Munich. I did not feel well; perhaps something like after-dissertation blues caught up with me. And K was working overtime every day. She works as a social worker for the city, within the department for homeless youth. Their situation is nightmarish at the moment. Most of them are locked down within camps, three to four sharing a room, and they face constant bullying by the cops.

We go out each day for an evening walk. The park is always empty; one hardly sees one or two couples hastening through the dusk. I admit that I underestimated the psychological effects of this life in a ghost town.

Now, you and your friends outlined a bunch of potential responses to Covid-19. I think the general options can be ordered as follows.

So, confronted with Covid-19, there are two basic options. The first is denial: we can deny that it exists, or, more likely, we could assert that it is nothing special.

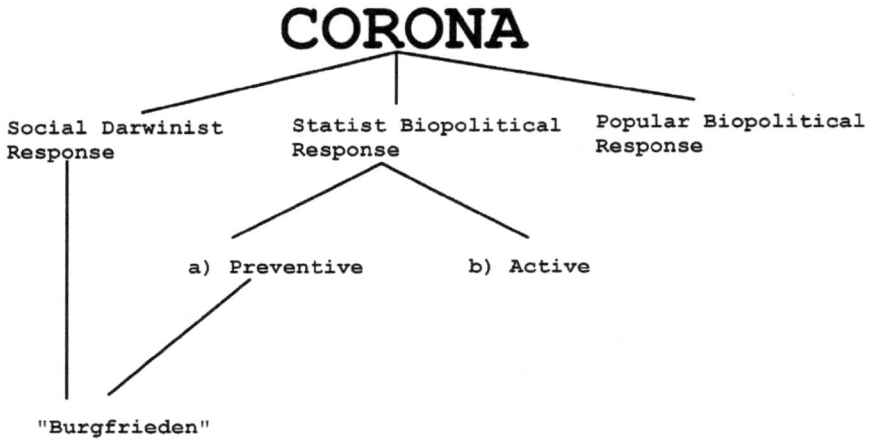

CORONA

Social Darwinist
Response

Statist Biopolitical
Response

Popular Biopolitical
Response

a) Preventive

b) Active

"Burgfrieden"

FIGURE 2.1

A mere flu. Let's put this response aside: nothing comes of it. The second and more meaningful option is to admit that Covid-19 is a predicament that demands a stringent response. To follow up on this second option, we can discern three possible responses, which I understand as: (1) Social Darwinist, (2) Statist Biopolitical, and (3) Popular Biopolitical.

There is some consanguinity between (1) and (2), but let me keep them distinct.

Response (1) essentially involves adapting Social Darwinist ideologies to the current situation. The epidemic is seen as a tool to purge society, be it that eco-fascists, like the allegedly 'fake' Extinction Rebellion posters announcing that the virus is a cure for global warming,[10] or be it that Covid-19 is understood as a means to 'cull the poor and weak' for the benefit of the economy.[11] The Social Darwinist response calls in general for doing nothing but accepting the pandemic as an unavoidable necessity. The reason offered for such inaction is that any action would in the end do too much harm; it is better to accept that a certain percentage of the people will die and look for opportunities in the likelihood that those would be the more 'unproductive' parts of society. This response goes so far that a governor of Texas calls for the self-sacrifice of the elderly in order to keep capitalism alive, according to report yesterday.[12] *Dulce et decorum est pro capitalia mori.*

The Social Darwinist response is represented by the extreme libertarian right, eco-fascists, and, partly, as it seems, by the Johnson and Putin administrations, which effectively allow Covid-19 space (even if they don't say it explicitly). At least Johnson has spoken of the necessity to build up herd immunity, which is tantamount to saying that the death of hundreds of thousands is an acceptable price for doing nothing.

Response (2), the State Biopolitical, can be divided into two sorts: (2a) preventive and (2b) active, in your terms, Suman.

The (2a) State Biopolitical response of preventive treatment is represented by most European countries, which try to implement measures of social engineering to prevent a serious outbreak. As you have outlined it, this response is connected to certain economic and political transformations which *might* take place now. I am not sure how to evaluate them, although I admit that at least in the education sector, this will result in swift and brutal digitalization. But it seems clear to me that (2a) and (1) take place under a common horizon. I propose to call this horizon after the German term for the national unity front at the beginning of WWI, 'Burgfrieden': the enemy, Covid-19, is at the gates, which is the reason a state of exception is considered necessary for response (2a) and is denied in response (1). Yet both (1) and (2a) share the idea that this crisis has to do with resilience, with strengthening the national body, the Volkskörper, either such that the nation will emerge stronger and more competitive after surviving the epidemic or such that the national body exhibits collective strength now. Both positions evoke notions of discipline, of national unity and action under contagious conditions and with regard to the global market conditions and the national market ratio. Left formations, having accepted response (2a), are giving up their distinctive programmes/platforms to join what Modi called the 'People's Curfew'.[13] Class conflict and critique of the government are suspended and refused as impeding the healing of the national body. In almost all cases, response (2a) comes with a strong emphasis on the individual. I should individuate to preserve my own body and thus help to render the national body resilient. The individual body thus becomes the site of a national politics of resilience; it consequently no longer belongs to me but to the state and the national unity front. Every transgression by the individual is thus a transgression that harms the resilience of the national collective and is accordingly punishable – a logic we are now familiar with in relation to smoking/taking drugs. Covid-19 has radicalized this tendency.

Response (2b) of strong State Biopolitical active treatment is perfectly boring. This is more or less the Chinese response as far as we know (and the response of some Asian countries and Cuba). I think of response (2b) as old-fashioned social-democratic. The state acts to fight for the life of its citizens by intervening heavily in the economic sphere. Here the individual body becomes estranged from the individual subject as well: the body of the sick is seen as a site to legitimize the state by fighting the virus. In a complete reversal of (2a), bodies should not be excluded and punished if they are deviant, but the deviant (sick) bodies should be (re-)included in the national unity body. In a kind of universalist act, the sick are seen as belonging to the national body. This position is perhaps disinvested from all desires of economic transformations but follows a strictly political logic, as its goal is to deliver a legitimization for the status quo and for the existing national project that adapts these responses.

Beyond these, a response (3) is thinkable: Popular Biopolitical. This is perhaps the weakest insofar as there are coherent formations that have adopted it (to my knowledge). The concrete forms that this response may take are diverse: from gangs in Brazil forcing people to stay home in favelas,[14] to Italian or Spanish unions organizing wildcat strikes.[15] Yet what characterizes (3) is that outside and sometimes against the sphere of state and capitalism, people organize to respond to Covid-19 contagions and to use this situation to realize long-term demands for a better life, higher wages, and so on. Response (3) might be a mixture of (1), (2a), and (2b). For example, when I go shopping for the elderly in my apartment block, I am somewhere between responses (1) and (2a). But this little act is determined to see Covid-19 as a moment of weakness of the ruling social formation and to accrue with other little acts so as to bring forth a combative position and organize a form of popular response. People use the virus, accepting its dangers to realize something. Memes circulate, as you might know, calling Covid-19 'Comrade Coronavirus'.[16]

My hope is with response (3). I hope to contribute to this position and feel that response (3) needs more theoretical work.

Notes

1 Robert J. Glass, Laura M. Glass, Walter E. Beyeler and H. Jason Min, 'Targeted social distancing designs for pandemic influenza', *Emerging Infectious Diseases Journal* 12:11, 2006, 1671–81, https://dx.doi.org/10.3201/eid1211.060255.
2 Homeland Security Council, US Government, *National Strategy for Pandemic Influenza: Implementation Plan* (2006), p. 14, www.cdc.gov/flu/pandemic-resources/pdf/pandemic-influenza-implementation.pdf (accessed 31 May 2020).
3 Karl Mannheim, *Essays on the Sociology of Culture* (Abingdon: Routledge, 1956), p. 210.
4 See Geoffrey Hunt, 'The development of the concept of civil society in Marx', *Journal of Political Thought* 8:2, Summer 1987, 263–76; William Niemi, 'Karl Marx's sociological theory of democracy: Civil society and political rights', *The Social Science Journal* 48:1, January 2011, 39–51, https://doi.org/10.1016/j.soscij.2010.07.002.
5 'Las favelas de Río, verdaderos caldos de cultivo para el coronavirus', *Agencia EFE*, 17 March 2020, www.efe.com/efe/america/sociedad/las-favelas-de-rio-verdaderos-caldos-cultivo-para-el-coronavirus/20000013-4198002; Ligia Guimarães, 'Favelas serão as grandes vítimas do coronavírus no Brasil, diz líder de Paraisópolis', *BBC Brazil*, 18 March 2020, www.bbc.com/portuguese/brasil-51954958 (accessed 29 May 2020). Officially the first case of Covid-19 was reported in Brazil on 26 February, but it is widely suspected that there were earlier cases.
6 Ricardo Della Coletta, 'Bolsonaro criticizes the closure of schools, attacks governors and blames the media in televised statement', *Folha de S.Paulo*, 25 March 2020, https://www1.folha.uol.com.br/internacional/en/brazil/2020/03/bolsonaro-criticizes-the-closure-of-schools-attacks-governors-and-blames-the-media-in-televised-statement.shtml; Tom Phillips, 'Bolsonaro says he "wouldn't feel anything" if infected with Covid-19 and attacks state lockdowns', *Guardian*, 25 March 2020, www.theguardian.com/world/2020/mar/25/bolsonaro-brazil-wouldnt-feel-anything-covid-19-attack-state-lockdowns (accessed 31 May 2020).
7 That Bolsonaro was effectively moving towards a coup by rousing his supporters to stop the Parliament and Supreme Court from functioning was widely suspected in news media by this date; see: Karlus Tamara, 'No, Bolsonaro's Brazil is not a dictatorship. It's worse', *Globe Post*, 4 March 2020, https://theglobepost.com/2020/03/04/bolsonaro-brazil/; Tom Phillips, 'Outrage as Jair Bolsonaro appears to endorse Brazil anti-democracy protests', *Guardian*, 26 February 2020, www.theguardian.com/world/2020/feb/26/jair-bolsonaro-brazil-anti-democracy-protests (accessed 29 May 2020).
8 Rede Globo is the largest commercial television network in Brazil, owned by the media conglomerate Grupo Globo. Established in 1965, its history involved working closely with the military dictatorship from 1964 to 1985. Friction between Bolsonaro and Rede Globo escalated particularly since October 2019, with broadcasts which suggested a link between the president's household and the 2018 murder of human rights activist

and Rio de Janeiro City Councillor Marielle Franco: see Andres Schipani and Bryan Harris, 'Bolsonaro rants at Brazil's top broadcaster on social media', *Financial Times,* 30 October 2019, www.ft.com/content/2ec18402-fb2a-11e9-a354-36acbbb0d9b6. Bolsonaro's hostility to mainstream media combined with his opposition to Covid-19 restrictions: see Tom Phillips, 'Brazil's Jair Bolsonaro says coronavirus crisis is a media trick', *Guardian*, 23 March 2020, www.theguardian.com/world/2020/mar/23/brazils-jair-bolsonaro-says-coronavirus-crisis-is-a-media-trick (accessed 29 May 2020).

 9 Akwugo Emejulu and Leah Bassel, 'The politics of exhaustion', *City*, 2020, DOI: 10.1080/13604813.2020.1739439.

10 'Coronavirus: Extinction rebellion distances itself from "fake posters"', *BBC*, 25 March 2020, www.bbc.com/news/uk-england-derbyshire-52039662 (accessed 29 May 2020).

11 Joe Roberts, 'Telegraph journalist says coronavirus "cull" of elderly could benefit economy', *Metro,* 11 March 2020, https://metro.co.uk/2020/03/11/telegraph-journalist-says-coronavirus-cull-elderly-benefit-economy-12383907/?ito=cbshare (accessed 29 May 2020).

12 Adrinna Rodriguez, 'Texas' lieutenant governor suggests grandparents are willing to die for US economy', *USA Today,* 24 March 2020, www.usatoday.com/story/news/nation/2020/03/24/covid-19-texas-official-suggests-elderly-willing-die-economy/2905990001/ (accessed 29 May 2020).

13 See the first intervention in the next chapter.

14 Ricardo Moraes, Debora Moreira and Rodrigo Viga Gaier, 'Gangs call curfews as coronavirus hits Rio favelas', *Reuters*, 25 March 2020, https://in.reuters.com/article/uk-health-coronavirus-brazil-favelas-fea/gangs-call-curfews-as-coronavirus-hits-rio-favelas-idINKBN21B3DP (accessed 29 May 2020).

15 Paola Tamma, 'Coronavirus sparks nationwide strikes in Italy', *Politico*, 13 March 2020, www.politico.eu/article/coronavirus-sparks-nationwide-strikes-in-italy/; Matt Day, Daniele Lepido, Helene Fouquet and Macarena Munoz Montijano, 'Coronavirus strikes at Amazon's operational heart: Its delivery machine', *Bloomberg*, 16 March 2020, www.bloomberg.com/news/articles/2020-03-16/coronavirus-strikes-at-amazon-s-operational-heart-its-delivery-machine (accessed 29 May 2020).

16 www.reddit.com/r/DankLeft/comments/fb6dem/comrade_coronavirus/ (accessed 29 May 2020).

3

LOCKDOWN

Summary: *As lockdowns start being announced in the various locations of the authors, this chapter begins by focusing on who takes responsibility for making announcements and imposing lockdowns and what effects the announcements are designed to have. The distinction between responsibility being taken by a specific person and by an officeholder (such as a head of state) is underlined. The ways in which messages to similar effect can be phrased to have distinct local connotations comes up. From there the chapter moves towards mulling the economic consequences of lockdown, in particular the part that the private sector – seemingly in the background at this juncture – could or should play.*

Suman Gupta (25 March 2020, Delhi, India)

Here's a thought from my friend Rekha:

> One thing I have observed [during the coronavirus lockdown in Delhi]: there is a lot of rallying around Modi now, even his diehard critics are listening to the eight pm broadcast by the PM. One colleague insisted that he was listening to the Prime Minister's speech and referring to a formal office, the individual occupying it a purely contingent circumstance.

This raises some interesting issues, which I try to consider here.

1   The observation is related specifically to the governmental regime led by Prime Minister Narendra Modi since 2014 but raises a question of general principle.

Let's start with the specific. Modi's government is ideologically religious (Hindu) nationalist and, for economic purposes, subscribes to privatization/disinvestment strategies for (putatively) development which end up benefitting the elites. In steps since 2014, it has fostered a brutally hostile environment for Muslims, Dalits, socialists, and liberal rationalists. Modi's alignment has been resoundingly successful in two general elections. Shortly before the coronavirus outbreak, there was concern about an economic downturn and high unemployment. Sustained and manifold protests were underway against a series of legislative moves and policy implementations which were recognized as motivated by Hindu nationalism even when thinly disguised by moral or legalistic rhetoric – and as undermining constitutional guarantees. A deadly communal riot had just taken place in the capital, Delhi.[1] There was also continuing evidence of strong support from, seemingly, the majority of the polity.

The general issue that arises in Rekha's observation is about the division of office (such as the position of prime minister of India) and officeholder (like Narendra Modi). It is exactly the sort of question that arises for an officeholder like Modi, because he (with his acolytes) tests received principles governing the office he holds. The same could be said of other heads of state: Donald Trump (United States), Recep Tayyib Erdogan (Turkey), Viktor Orbán (Hungary), Rodrigo Duterte (Philippines), Jair Bolsonaro (Brazil), and others.

2   The challenging issue of clarifying the separation of office and officeholder, especially at the top of a political formation, involves several factors.

   a   In any modern institutional setting, the office is positioned in relation to other offices within and outside the institution and with regard to the overall purpose of the institution. This positioning follows a purposive institutional rationale. Max Weber's outline of bureaucratic order gives an account of this institutional rationale.[2] Very briefly, what it amounts to is that the bureaucratic ordering includes arrangements for separating officeholder and office by putting (legally enjoined or good practice) limits on the interference of the officeholder's personal interests and biases, such that the respective parts of other offices are best utilized and the overall purpose of the institution is best served.

   b   However, this institutional rationale does maintain space for the officeholder as such, as a person (or personality). The limitations in question are not such as remove choices from officeholders, especially in their upper rungs. The officeholder has choices and prerogatives, and how those are exercised in given contexts is expressive of the particular officeholder. Thus, appointments are cognizant of officeholders' personalities and opinions; elections as appointment processes are obviously so. Prerogatives of office are also more or less flexible; they can be strictly limited by law or flexible according to convention or need. That also offers choice to officeholders.

c Insofar as large political institutions go – like the business of government in formal democracies – choice is imbued in the office itself. Multiparty politics in elective and parliamentary systems, separated from the judiciary, give considerable flexibility in the exercise and determination of choices and therefore in the expression of the officeholder's proclivities in the functioning of office.

d Not everything of an officeholder's exercising of an office can be anticipated and fixed by tenet or principle; in fact, quite a lot can't. There are numerous nuances which might be outside the scope of bureaucratic ordering – such as subtleties of expression, manner, behaviour, character, and so on which give a distinctive flavour to a particular officeholder's functioning in an office.

3 The coronavirus outbreak and the need for preventive treatment is not a matter of political choice. The denial for the need of such treatment might show personal stupidity; the acceptance and sensible implementation thereof is a matter of evidence and reasoning for an inevitable course rather than a political choice.

So, this is not a political choice, but its implementation is a responsibility of government, and the officeholders in the government have appeared as such by exercising political choices. However, given that this is not a political choice, it is reasonable to take cognizance of the office responsible for its implementation in terms of its pure bureaucratically rationalized position – irrespective of the political choices made by the officeholders in other circumstances.

So, it is reasonable to attend seriously to Modi in terms of his office as prime minister insofar as that bears upon preventive treatment of coronavirus (social distancing, etc.), irrespective of how reprehensible the officeholder Modi's political record and ideological inclinations might seem to some.

4 To that extent, it is reasonable. But there is a further consideration. In fulfilling the responsibility of his office as prime minister to implement a measure which is not a political choice, is officeholder Modi nevertheless imbuing that measure with his political inclinations? As someone at odds with Modi's politics, I may attend to him seriously and compliantly as prime minister responsible for measures to deal with the coronavirus outbreak and yet be troubled by some ideological nuance that he manages to imbue into the process. Is that the case in this instance?

I did find myself troubled in that way. In fact, like Rekha's colleague, the diehard critic of Modi, who listened to his speeches on the coronavirus lockdowns, so did I and attentively. In substance, the measures he declared seem harsh but on the whole necessary in India at present.

In style there was something else – small things, but troubling. I have in mind rhetorical turns in his speeches on 19 March and 24 March 2020. In both, he seemed inordinately fond of declaring curfews rather than lockdowns.

> Today, I request my fellow citizens for support on one more issue, that of people's curfew. People's curfew [Janata curfew] means a curfew imposed for the people, by the people, on the people themselves. (19 March)[3]

> All the States in the country, all the Union Territories, each district, each municipality, each village, each locality is being put under lockdown.
> This is like a curfew only.
> This will be a few levels more than Janata-Curfew, and also stricter. (24 March)[4]

It might be fortuitous that such declarations come shortly after he had declared an indefinite curfew in Kashmir following an act of state (withdrawal of Article 370), in the midst of an unexceptional situation, amidst reasonable social stability, on 5 August 2019[5] – possibly the first in the country post-independence to be announced without significant unrest on the ground or a declaration of exception to explain it. So, suddenly, people going about their everyday lives in a region found themselves under curfew, unable to leave their homes, get on the Internet, move round the city freely, or leave the region, with military barricades and personnel all around – a proper curfew in the way that term has been understood so far.

In these speeches, the Janata (people's) Curfew that Modi has been harping about has something out of joint in it. It seems to make curfews a democratic responsibility and medicine (for the people, by the people, on the people themselves); it sugar-coats coercive acts of state which have been used in increasingly suspect ways of late. At the same time, it effectively connects the withdrawal of the right to assemblage of more than five or three people due to the coronavirus outbreak to a kind of criminal notion of 'unlawful assembly'. In law, Section 141 of the Indian Penal Code makes this clear, where such assembly is understood as designed, 'To overawe by criminal force, or show of criminal force', or 'To resist the execution of any law, or of any legal process', or 'To commit any mischief or criminal trespass, or other offence', and so on. Protecting people from disease and containing antisocial activity seem to become the same sort of thing. To my mind, there is also something out of joint in Modi's calling for a ritual collective expression of gratitude to essential workers during the coronavirus. It seemed much like a kind of religious ritual – or a motivational celebration, which isn't much different from a religious ritual. Neighbours where I am living responded spiritedly to the call, and, according to news reports, a festive spirit took over the whole country at that time. At the least, apart from showing the gratitude of the people for essential workers, it showed something of Modi's populist power and ability to get a population dancing to his tune. Modi is a wordsmith; he knows the measured nuances of the words he chooses.

Milena Katsarska (25 March 2020, Plovdiv, Bulgaria)

I think that the qualifications and cautionary observations about 'People's Curfew' and 'unlawful assembly' are important. These can be linked to various proclamations which seem to be received as referring to neutral non-political issues (relevant across different nation-states) but which are, in fact, rendered deeply political and suspect when issued by a specific person holding an office in a specific context. A case in point are such proclamations by Viktor Orbán in Hungary,[6] from where I returned just as the lockdown began. This is not necessarily a matter solely of reframing, that is, focalizing one context (or displacing it) from a broader one. It isn't merely a matter of shifting the perspective from the overall measures for a peculiar medical emergency to placing those measures within a narrower but longer chain of authoritarian, xenophobic, or undemocratic measures. If one combs through linguistic expressions used in proclamations in different countries by different leaders, one might actually find slight but locally telling variations of vocabulary. The deployment of any statement as addressed to any polity speaks to that polity within the discourse flow addressed to that polity for a chunk of time (as far as recent memory goes).

In this respect, the Bulgarian case – as perhaps in some other countries (?) – is slightly different. This was evident the moment a 'crisis HQ' was set up and a spokesperson other than the head of state/ministers/political spokespersons was fronted to publicly announce decisions regarding Covid-19. This is playing out interestingly these days, with crisis boss General/Surgeon Mutafchiyski announcing measures in a moderate tone, always stepping aside to give the floor to this or that medical expert when a question calls for it. Prime Minister Borisov, who has tended to be in the limelight for all public affairs for a longish time, is now less prominently featured in the media. Laws are being drafted or vehemently debated in Parliamentary halls. Neither Prime Minister Borisov nor President Radev is actually the one giving the key messages for Covid-19. This could well be a sensible ploy, that is, one that reduces political readings/interpretations. That is not to say that there aren't any. But it is a curious situation. It creates a different dynamic from Orbán's in Hungary, Trump's in the United States, or Modi's in India. I wonder which countries go along with a head of state and which have wheeled out a specially appointed crisis HQ leader as the top message sender on 'emergency measures'.

Peter H. Tu (26 March 2020, Niskayuna, New York State, United States)

They say that the people with the least probability of ever changing their minds are the intellectuals. When presented with conflicting evidence, 99% of our mental energy goes into building arguments as to why such data actually supports our personal convictions as opposed to even considering the possibility that we might be wrong. From time to time, I find myself wondering if a Democrat had suggested a new policy instead of a Republican, would I have been so hostile to it. . . . Modi is most certainly an unsavoury character, but he does hold the office which from time to time needs to perform certain functions in order for the system to function.

From my side, I wish that I had such dilemmas. Everything that comes out of Trump's mouth feels untrustworthy. . . . He is currently at war with Andrew Cuomo (governor of New York) because Cuomo's daily briefings come off like a suave fireside chat, making Trump look like a hesitant novice (Mario Cuomo, Andrew's father, was one of the great orators of his time). One of the problems is that Trump's brand of identity politics implies that in spite of his lack of knowledge, he should in no way have his actions restricted or curtailed by experts. He fears that any capitulation to expertise will result in his base losing faith. Up until now, he has gotten away with this:

Experts:	You can't threaten North Korea with nuclear annihilation.
Trump:	Oh yes, I can, just watch me.
Experts:	You can't renege on the Iran deal.
Trump:	Oh yes, I can, just watch me.
Experts:	You can't pull out of the climate change accords.
Trump:	Oh yes, I can, just watch me.
Experts:	You need to have a country-wide shutdown now.
Trump:	No, I don't.
Experts:	You need to force industry to build the necessary supplies and have the federal government distribute it.
Trump:	No, I don't.

Trump now predicts that this will all be over by Easter Sunday.[7] Fox News continues to promote its 'it's all a liberal hoax meant to make Trump look bad' arguments. It claims that liberals are intentionally tanking the economy to hurt Trump. While the federal government fails to jump in and orchestrate the procurement and distribution of medical materials, a number of Republican governors are holding his line. In Mississippi, local mayors are issuing lockdown orders; however, Governor Tate Reeves, who states that 'Mississippi's never going to be China!', has overturned all these orders, and now everyone has to go back to work, can go to restaurants and live as if nothing is going on.[8] Meanwhile, Louisiana (the state next to Mississippi) has the fastest increasing death-rate in the world, which has been attributed to the decision not to stop Mardi Gras a few weeks ago. Even Boris Johnson, who seemed to be attracted to Trump's thumbing his nose at experts in a Brexity-throw-caution-to-the-wind kind of way, seems to have recently seen the light.

Peter H. Tu (29 March 2020, Niskayuna, New York State, United States)

As I hit day 14 of sheltering-in-place, I have shifted metaphors. I started with the zombie classic *Walking Dead*. That's mostly because of the fear of interacting with strangers and the empty shelves at the grocery stores. Since then, I have decided that this is more like being on a space ship that has crash landed on an inhospitable planet, much like the movie *The Martian* (which, if you have not seen it yet, is really quite good). The house has taken on a pod-like feeling. In my basement, I can ride my stationary bike; lift weights; play ping-pong, pool, and foosball (a kind of soccer game popular in the pubs). In my living room, I have my television as well as my make-shift office. Our freezer has all sorts of frozen foods that feel like things astronauts would eat. I can take the dog out for walks around the block, but there is a sense of 'suiting up' whenever I go outside and decontamination when I return – it is like being on a kind of space-walk of sorts. My front porch also has an element of seeing the natural world from a distance, kind of like a space deck. When neighbors go by, we chat but from opposite sides of the street. More and more I have to ration my options for variety. I know that if I use the basement too much, I will soon grow bored of it. I have even gotten to the point where I start to look forward to a scheduled teleconference just so I can hear a new voice from time to time.

I am scheduled to go to the doctor's on Thursday this week; I had some mild surgery a few weeks ago – nothing serious – and now I need to have the stitches removed. It will be my first outing. In a strange way, I am looking forward to it. On the bright side, the nerve damage that I suffered last year seems to have fully healed, and I no longer have to wear an eye patch. I had hoped to restart my tennis game, but all the courts have been closed.

Suman Gupta (1 April 2020, Delhi, India)

As the Covid-19 lockdowns are implemented across the world, the hands of government seem to hold and dispense everything. Government leaders are centre stage, public money is being dispensed to protect the threatened public, publicly funded health and other essential workers are prominently on the frontline. We might understandably ask: what is happening with the profit-making private sector?

There's a top-down view of how the Covid-19 measures are turning out for the global economy. IMF Managing Director Kristalina Georgieva said in a press briefing of 27 March:

> It is now clear that we have entered a recession – as bad as or worse than in 2009. We do project recovery in 2021 – in fact there may be a sizeable

rebound, but only if we succeed with containing the virus – everywhere – and prevent liquidity problems from becoming a solvency issue. A key concern about a long-lasting impact of the sudden stop of the world economy is the risk of a wave of bankruptcies and layoffs that not only can undermine the recovery but can erode the fabric of our societies.[9]

It might be inferred that this is as bad for businesses as for individual livelihoods and prospects. The governmental apparatus of the publicly funded sector is stepping in where the profit-making private sector and private lives are beleaguered; recovery depends upon that. After that there might be a great return to normalcy – what sort of normalcy, though?

The reference to the recession of 2009 is not innocent. Back in 2014–2016, I participated in a project on the financial crisis from 2007–8 onwards in Europe with colleagues from the United Kingdom, Ireland, Greece, Cyprus, Bulgaria, and elsewhere. We were trying to determine how that recession – and the consequent austerity policies, unemployment, decimation of publicly funded services – was being understood at ground level. We felt that though the deleterious effects of the crisis were felt most painfully at the ground level of work and livelihoods, governmental and media communications were overwhelmingly dominated by Big Players: mainly, global financial organizations and governments. It wasn't at all clear whether these Big Players were avid collaborators or mildly at odds; it was clear that they weren't adversaries. The mendacity and rapacity of very large financial organizations had produced this crisis, but the governments seemed to think the world couldn't do without them and bailed out the biggest with huge pay-outs of public money – at the expense of the publicly funded sector, not to speak of the livelihoods and securities of the less affluent. The bailed-out organizations were in principle nationalized but remained legally private, and most were able to pay off their debts to the public at below-market interest rates or even with discounts. The corrupt practices and the venal agencies which had caused the crisis largely continued undeterred. It seemed that governments exist to protect the most weighty of the profit-making private sector at the expense of the publicly funded sector, and the health of society depends upon governments working hand in hand with the former so that they can carry on innovating, being efficient, capturing gigantic market shares, providing benefits for profits, marketizing welfare, minimizing the public sector, making minimal (at times undetectable) proportional tax contributions . . . and being corrupt. Indeed, for around four decades preceding the 2009 recession, that had been the mantra (with the corruption bit left out) which was drilled unceasingly into the hive-mind of the capitalist world.

Fast forward to 2020 March, and no one in government is calling upon the profit-making private sector to save the day. Rather governments are now apparently mainly wheeling out the long-beleaguered and much-whittled publicly funded services to save the world and are making direct investments of public money to the public which gave it to the government in the first place. There seems to be no talk of the 'entrepreneurial energy and efficiency', 'public-private partnerships', and 'corporate social responsibility' which we have grown accustomed to. Some high-profile corporations are doing what seem like low-key charity work out of profitless goodness. Otherwise, it seems that the profit-making private sector is as vulnerable to Covid-19 as human bodies. Here's something of a volte face.

Among those who have long felt that too much of the publicly funded sector has been eroded over the years, the optimistic find a sliver of hope for the future in this unusual turn. The cynical among them cannot help detecting an ironic chime in the motivational bells being rung for the public sector by governments. But what about the private sector?

A few ancillary questions come to mind to begin exploring this.

To pose these questions, some distinctions are expedient. Of course 'profit-making private sector' is too sweeping a term and 'publicly funded sector' too pat a term as the counterpart. Further distinctions need to be kept in mind, at three levels. First, there are big businesses (national, multinational, and global corporations) and there are 'micro-, small- and medium-sized enterprises' (MSMEs). Second, there are service-providing and manufacturing businesses. Third, there are formal and informal – which correspond to regulated and unregulated – businesses. Naturally these distinctions overlap variously, even counterintuitively. Big businesses could have significant informal/unregulated activity (such as shadow banking); a single business operation could incorporate all those polarities and combine them variously; MSMEs defined by workforce could have large turnovers and operate at a global scale; under current regulations in various countries, profit-making businesses can take advantage of investments and tax breaks for public services; and so on. So, questions:

1   Which large profit-making businesses may have gained from the Covid-19 lockdowns? As a plausible guess, volumes of uptake on online activity have gone up: financial, retailing, contracting, recording, conferencing, networking, designing, and other services would have made a step change in concentrating on online and telecom facilities. At bottom, these facilities are provided by a handful of global megacorporations (Google, Amazon, Facebook, Microsoft, Visa, MasterCard, Tencent, Alibaba, Baidu, PayPal, Netflix, AT&T, China Mobile, Verizon, and a few more hold a large share of the market). On the one hand, I am aware of no reduction in their service charges, so presumably with increased volumes of uptake, their profit margins would have increased. On the other hand, their corporate customer base (companies in difficulty due to Covid-19) may have diminished a bit, which might adversely affect profits – but I doubt it. Pharmaceutical and healthcare equipment providers are another area of profit-making activity that have probably benefitted, as variously observed previously.

2   To what degree have businesses which have benefitted from the Covid-19 lockdowns meant that other businesses have lost out? In an obvious way, big online retailers are likely to have gained by the curtailment of small – especially localized – retailing. As a guess, it seems likely that MSMEs would have lost

out to big business in the service sector, and manufacturing may have taken a downturn relative to services.

3   To what extent has the government's public money expenditure on managing the Covid-19 crisis been used for direct public services or been sieved through profit-making businesses (i.e. have covered both their profits and the service costs)? That depends greatly on how much of the apparently publicly funded sector is covertly privately operated (outsourced or tendered out). It also depends significantly upon how far governments, having watered down public capacities, are now consumers of the profit-making private sector for essential goods and services to battle the pandemic – and on what terms. Are they making good deals on behalf of their stricken populations with those populations' money?

4   How much of the public expenditures announced for bailouts and handouts reached the hands of individuals and households in need, how much was creamed off by businesses administering them, and how much has been directed towards sustaining businesses in danger of going under? For the last, importantly, what are the conditions of these bailouts? Are they like the bailouts given to corrupt financial sector organizations in the 2009 crisis? These might sound like several questions but are parts of one issue.

5   To what extent has the private sector spent on their 'corporate social responsibility' without the condition of direct profits and relative to their profits? This could include expenditure in alleviating some aspect of the crisis without making a profit other than indirectly through, say, profile raising. Is that a larger proportion of their profits than usual? Has it happened at all? Since not much has been heard of it, it is perhaps limited – not much profile raising is happening at the moment.

Are there other questions along these lines?

Depending on the answers, it might turn out that the Covid-19 crisis has already become the perfect neoliberal juncture in which governments are fronting and protecting big business interests so blandly that the latter have become invisible . . . and are making or are set to make a killing.

Milena Katsarska (1 April 2020, Plovdiv, Bulgaria)

Will try to think of other big-scale questions because the ones I was thinking about seem to be in subdivisions of one or several of these.

Earlier I had mentioned the math for the 'generous promise' of the government to cover 60% of salaries in 'affected businesses'. Let me go back to it.

Let's leave aside two things, important as they are: (1) what parameters will qualify you as 'an affected business' and (2) the disparity between declared/registered salaries and the actual money you get paid a month. To explain the latter: it is a standard practice that businesses declare a lower salary on which social securities and health insurance are paid and retirement pay is calculated and add something extra for the worker in 'the gray area of the economy'. It is supposed that smaller businesses resort to this somewhat shady practice because the bigger ones can afford not to, though I am not sure. But that's neither here nor there. The big noise in Bulgarian government and business circles now is that the promised 60% coverage is too small because the employer still has to pay the dues for social security and taxation. So, the most optimistic estimate is that in real terms, this in fact amounts to 23% covered by the government, while in the case of R's small business, for instance, this will mean a 10% state subsidy of the three salaries he is to provide for these months – provided the business had never resorted to declaring 'unpaid leave' for its workers for the past 12 months (how many of those and of what length, huh?). However, there are some businesses whose profits makes it easy peasy for them to cover several months of salaries even without any actual productivity.

Then there is the murky division of private/public hospitals in Bulgaria (I heard the number 380 for hospitals that we have here, without specifics as to how many fall into each category), whereby private hospitals have the greater share of the 'market' that is insured by the healthcare fund. That is, private hospitals can also (and do) claim healthcare system subsidies/payments. In other words, I can go into a private hospital to do what is necessary to be done to me and that will be covered by my state-paid social/healthcare plan. I will not be considered a 'private patient', paying out of my own pocket, although I might be asked to 'cover the difference' if the service's cost exceeds the cap on coverage by the public sector. I don't understand how this can be a rational arrangement between public and private sectors; it seems to me as if it is a mechanism for public funds not to be invested in the public sector but to feed the private sector.

Going into further Bulgarian specifics, I am curious about the current deals that the biggest private pharmaceutical company Sopharma is striking these days. The top-dog owner reputedly operates on a big scale, having acquired the former state enterprise for a pittance back in the late 1990s. He also owns arguably the most high-tech private hospital in Sofia, as well as several other specialized hospitals scattered in smaller, nondescript towns. The news mentioned almost in passing that Sopharma has begun local production of hydroxychloroquine,[10] the current rage, commissioned by the government. That was it, a mention in passing, for something that is probably huge.

Notes

1 Jeffrey Gettleman, Suhasini Raj and Sameer Yassir, 'The roots of the Delhi riots: A fiery speech and an ultimatum', *New York Times*, 26 February 2020, www.nytimes. com/2020/02/26/world/asia/delhi-riots-kapil-mishra.html (accessed 29 May 2020); Hannah Ellis-Petersen, 'Inside Delhi: Beaten, lynched and burnt alive', *Guardian*, 1 March 2020, www.theguardian.com/world/2020/mar/01/india-delhi-after-hindu-mob-riot-religious-hatred-nationalists (accessed 29 May 2020).
2 Max Weber, *Economy and Society: An Outline of Interpretive Sociology* (Berkeley CA: University of California Press, 1978 [1922]), Ch.11.

3 Narendra Modi, 'Address to the nation', 19 March 2020, English transcript, www.narendramodi.in/text-of-prime-minister-narendra-modi-s-address-to-the-nation-on-combating-covid-19-548861 (accessed 31 May 2020).

4 Narendra Modi, 'Address to the nation', 24 March 2020, English transcript, www.narendramodi.in/text-of-prime-minister-narendra-modi-s-address-to-the-nation-on-vital-aspects-relating-to-the-menace-of-covid-19-548941 (accessed 31 May 2020).

5 For different accounts of this curfew, see: Ayjaz Wani, 'Life in Kashmir after Article 370', *Observer Research Foundation Special Report No.99*, 28 January 2020, www.orfonline.org/research/life-in-kashmir-after-article-370-60785/; International Federation for Human Rights, 'Update on human rights violations in Indian-administered Jammu & Kashmir six months on', 5 February 2020, www.fidh.org/IMG/pdf/20200205_india_kashmir_bp_en.pdf; Ather Zia, 'The haunting specter of Hindu ethnonationalist-neocolonial development in the Indian occupied Kashmir', *Development* 63, 2020, 60–66, https://doi.org/10.1057/s41301-020-00234-4 (accessed 29 May 2020).

6 'Hungary's Orban blames foreigners, migration for coronavirus spread', *France 24*, 13 March 2020, www.france24.com/en/20200313-hungary-s-pm-orban-blames-foreign-students-migration-for-coronavirus-spread; 'Hungarian PM Orban insists on special powers to handle virus crisis, mulls lockdown', *Reuters*, 23 March 2020, https://in.reuters.com/article/health-coronavirus-hungary-lockdown/hungarian-pm-orban-insists-on-special-powers-to-handle-virus-crisis-mulls-lockdown-idINKBN21A2F2 (accessed 29 May 2020).

7 Kevin Liptak, Maegan Vazquez, Nick Valencia and Jim Acosta, 'Trump says he wants the country 'opened up and just raring to go by Easter,' despite health experts' warnings', *CNN*, 25 March 2020, https://edition.cnn.com/2020/03/24/politics/trump-easter-economy-coronavirus/index.html (accessed 29 May 2020).

8 Nick Judin, 'Governor rejects state lockdown for COVID-19: "Mississippi's never going to be China"', *Jackson Free Press*, 23 March 2020, www.jacksonfreepress.com/photos/2020/mar/23/36424/ (accessed 29 May 2020).

9 'Opening remarks at a press briefing by Kristalina Georgieva following a conference call of the international monetary and financial committee (IMFC)', *International Monetary Fund*, 27 March 2020, www.imf.org/en/News/Articles/2020/03/27/sp032720-opening-remarks-at-press-briefing-following-imfc-conference-call (accessed 30 May 2020).

10 The news about a prospective government order, following negotiations, for the production of chloroquine was reported in the morning briefings in connection with a donation on behalf of Sopharma to hospitals in Sofia: first to the amount of 350,000 BGN in 'Премиерът: Сервитьори, бармани и пикола временно да минат към социалната система, вместо да си седят вкъщи', *TrafficNews*, 22 March 2020, https://trafficnews.bg/obshtestvo/premierat-servityori-barmani-i-pikola-vremenno-da-minat-kam-172991/. Later there was a report with a reference to 33,000 packages of quinine made available at the Military Medical Academy as a result from a donation from Sopharma: '25 нови случая на коронавирус, заразата стигна Силистра', *DarikNews.bg*, 31 March 2020, https://dariknews.bg/novini/bylgariia/25-novi-sluchaia-na-koronavirus-zarazata-stigna-silistra-2219452. In early April, Minister of Health Ananiev reported on an agreement 'reached between Sopharma and the government for the production of Analgin-Chinin', see: 'Има алгоритми за лечение с хлорохин', *Clinica.bg*, 13 April 2020, https://clinica.bg/11735-Ima-algoritmi-za-lechenie-s-hlorohin (accessed 31 May 2020).

4

SUSPENSION OF POLITICS

Summary: *As life under lockdown settles, the usual business of politics seems to be overtaken by a localized, narrow, and domestic sense of political interests anchored to the apolitical fact of Covid-19. Starting with this observation, this chapter offers glimpses of the routine, trivial, and farcical political performances that took place. Motivational actions played a forgettable part at the time. A great burgeoning of conspiracy theories was a notable if predictable feature at this juncture. The reactions of anti-vaccination conspiracy theorists, whose convictions might be expected to have taken a hit, are outlined.*

Suman Gupta (3 April 2020, Delhi, India)

Once the shock of suddenly finding oneself locked down and the novelty of daily locked-down life wear off a bit, a sort of numbed routine sets in. Party or partisan politics, debates or doubts on a range of issues in the usual way seem a matter of indifference at ground level – politics is suspended. This state of suspended politics has a distinctive political character.

From the top, this suspension of politics is variously expressed.

I was watching Jeremy Corbyn's last appearance as leader of the opposition during the UK parliamentary PM's questions on BBC World a few days back.[1] The honourable members were seated at a safe distance from each other in the House of Commons. Corbyn was asking some tough questions about measures taken for workers whose livelihoods are threatened, and Johnson was sitting smirking and saying something cutting. Corbyn reprimanded him. 'This is no time for levity,' he observed, and continued pushing his point. Then Johnson stood up and, incredibly, said something like, 'He's quite right, this is not the time for levity'. In fact, he said

'He's quite right' *twice* in the midst of Corbyn's questioning. Perhaps the profound significance of this moment of accord, albeit at the last gasp of Corbyn's place on the front benches, escaped none. Normal politics has been suspended. No longer do Johnson and Corbyn have to slag each other off as a matter of principle and get Brexit done or undone. Shortly afterwards, Johnson announced that he too had been infected, but not debilitated, by the dreaded virus.

Not long after – today, in fact – I watched the honourable Narendra Modi's much publicized morning address to the Indian people.[2] No concession to presenting facts about or policies, plans, strategies to counter the contagion in this; its main point was asking the people of India to switch off their electric lights, step out on their front yards or balconies, light a candle or flash a torchlight or mobile flashlight, on 5 April at 9 pm for nine minutes. I think most of the people of India will actually do it, just as most obeyed when he called upon them to play gongs and bells and clap on their balconies at 5 pm on 22 March, the day of the 'Janata Curfew'. Modi has clearly decided that this is no time for politics in the usual way, that the common *janata* doesn't need to be burdened with arguments and explanations: this is a time for ritual and farce.

The suspension of politics in the usual way takes various forms at the top. The politics of the suspension of politics as viewed from below has some common descriptive features.

1   All matters of political moment are reorganized around a single apolitical force – an exponentially contagious virus without cure or vaccine. No ideology or political agency can be conferred on Covid-19; it's 'an act of god' in the legal sense, a *force majeure* insurance matter; none can be held responsible. (The pious may take a different view, claim that the Flood or the Great Turtle's tectonic movements were also *force majeure*, but let's put such nonsense aside for a while.) From a political perspective, there's a certain immovable quality about this apolitical reference point. All politics becomes conditional to it or immaterial beside it. If a question of politics comes up, such as support for one or another political party in forthcoming elections, it is regarded as a matter of indifference beside the absolute of the Covid-19 condition. Or else such a question, to do perhaps with inequality or nationalism or the climate crisis, becomes conditional – what do the Covid-19 outbreak and global lockdowns mean for that? How are those issues affected?

2   However, the numbed indifference or mild conditional interest is at the same time a particular sort of juncture – transient, temporary, for a while but not too long (hopefully). It is a righteous numbness, because the suspension of politics at this juncture is no more than a deferral in favour of something more significant. The importance of political life is not wholly eschewed; it is postponed for a greater-than-political, an apolitical, *ethical* juncture. In the midst of this juncture, talking about politics in the usual way – important as that may be – is a kind of obscenity or crassness. That is best postponed while we acknowledge our dutiful assent to this ethical juncture and wait for it to pass.

3 The measure of this ethical juncture is objectively signified by the burgeoning presence of Covid-19, in constantly updated numbers of confirmed cases and deaths – globally and country by country and particularly the country one is locked in. The emotional investments made by those contemplating these numbers at ground level are powerful, barely describable. On the one hand, they threaten a constant defeat – they fascinate by their expression of speed and voracity. On the other hand, they offer the continuous possibility of victory – the number-lines flatten a bit somewhere, dip there, rise precipitously towards a crest, after which there can only be a trough. On the third hand, those numbers suggest a target, an extraordinary zero point of the elimination of Covid-19 in the fullness of time, something to strive towards as one may strive for perfection. On the fourth hand (we all have four arms), those numbers instil a sense of continuity, a kind of reconciliation with the possibility of never talking to anyone again except at several arms' length and never visiting another city or country again or having a leisurely meal in a restaurant before a concert.

4 In the ethical juncture of suspended politics, which is only for a while, but perhaps for a very long while as the numbers roll, the remnant of political life shrinks into mundaneness and little worlds. The performance of the ethical juncture and suspended politics at ground level takes the form of an intense and virtuous concentration of small doings, in the online office and the domestic niche. Many of my friends are teachers who have moved from real to online classrooms (for a while, maybe forever). They teach online with a sense of mission that their real classrooms seldom witnessed (or at the least, so one gathers). Keeping on top of administrative chores becomes a moral responsibility. Deference to managers' and colleagues' rightful prerogatives, consideration for clients who are vulnerable in these difficult times – these assume a luminous significance where otherwise all those professional attitudes, when casually struck, were bread and butter. The main focus of political economy is the domestic unit, a condensation of locale, nation, and globe now: are any in the family showing symptoms? Is there enough food in the store? Are there enough sanitizers and toilet paper rolls? How is the day divided for you? What's for entertainment and exercise? . . .

Fabio Akcelrud Durão (3 April 2020, São Carlos, São Paulo State, Brazil)

In Brazil, the situation is somewhat different; we have the only president in the world who is rejecting the virus as a threat.[3] Bolsonaro's health minister Luiz Mandetta is dealing with Covid-19 as any reasonable person would (only more incompetently), while Bolsonaro accuses him every day.[4] So now you have a division between the full political spectrum on the one hand and Bolsonaro and his support group on the other, arguing that the virus is at bottom harmless and that people should immediately go back to work.

According to the last poll (today), Bolsonaro still has 28% approval rating,[5] which is enough not to be removed from office if his supporters are vocal about it. Bolsonaro has only one card to play, inducing chaos (either because people can't eat; because they can't work; or because they all went to the streets, got sick, and are dying in the open) so that he can stage a coup. On yet another (fifth) hand, Bolsonaro's vice president Hamilton Mourão is a general with no party support, though he seems at present to ensure military support. So the conclusion seems to be that in one way or another, we are heading here for a moment of great instability after the quarantine is over. I'll let you know, of course, if I survive . . .

Peter H. Tu (4 April 2020, Niskayuna, New York State, United States)

Suman, this story has played out many times before. In the US, 9–11 and Katrina (the hurricane that struck New Orleans, killing thousands) come to mind. Politically speaking, the George W. Bush administration was lauded for its response to 9–11 but criticized for Katrina. As you say, the winning formula seems to be quite simple: Leader X sets up a podium at or near the epicenter – thanks the first responders for their heroism (which is, of course, warranted), declares that this is no time for politics and that the nation must now come together. Thus Bush got re-elected in 2004 and New York's mayor during 9–11, Rudy Giuliani, was affectionately dubbed 'America's mayor'. This formula is so simple that just about any leader who follows this recipe will observe a significant bounce in their approval ratings.

However, the political winds can go south pretty fast. In Canada, any popular mayor is almost guaranteed to lose an election if, after a significant snowfall, they fail to clear the streets in a timely manner. For this reason, in northern climates, snow removal budgets are always the last thing to be cut, even during periods of austerity. This is odd, given the fact that snow does melt – you just have to be patient. . . . While Bush's response to 9–11 probably got him re-elected in 2004, his approval ratings took a nose dive after his handling of Katrina (2005) was widely criticized. Bush had assigned Michael Brown to be the head of FEMA. Mr. Brown's main credential was that he was commissioner of the International Arabian Horse Association for nine years. What is so baffling is that Trump's handling of Covid-19 makes Katrina look like a masterclass in logistics and professionalism and yet his approval ratings continue to not only hold but rise.

In my spare time, I have been working on modifying an old joke that I like to tell. It goes something like this.

An engineer, a physicist, and a human resources manager (HRM) were stuck on a tropical island with only a single can of beans. The three castaways set up camp on the beach and were discussing how they might get at their one and only food source. The engineer declared that she has an idea. She suggested that they use the engineer's favorite device – the lever. She proposed that a large stick be tied to a sturdy rock (the fulcrum) and that the short end of the stick be placed on top of the can. By elevating the long end of the stick, the resulting external pressure will crush the can, thus releasing its contents. The physicist and the HRM demurred. The physicist pointed out that this uncontrolled approach will result in the beans being exposed to the sand rendering them inedible. The engineer acknowledged their concerns. The physicist then declared that he had a thought. He proposed that they search for a giant clam shell. His idea was that the shape of such mollusc domiciles are roughly parabolic. They can then position the shell so that the sun's rays are focused on the can. The temperature will rise. The resulting internal pressure will cause a rupturing of the vessel. While the engineer recognized the elegance of this solution, she was quick to point out that an exploding can of beans was even more problematic than crushing it. . . . It was at this point that the HRM raised his hand. Both the engineer and the physicist were sceptical but reluctantly agreed to hear the HRM out. The HRM said: 'Why don't we simply talk to a real-estate developer – or better yet, ask his son-in-law?'

Coming up on day 21 of shelter-in-place . . .

Sebastian Schuller (5 April 2020, Munich, Germany)

On Covid-19 and numbness: Suman, I find your observations convincing but disheartening. And I am really driven, maybe even against my better judgement, to put a small spark of hope – which may start a prairie fire! – in it.

It's all right, what you write: the world has collapsed and is atomized into many little worlds. And I agree. Political discourse has become void at this point. Declarations by left groups circulating variously in social networks seem, even if they meet the situation, completely outlandish. Political action is not possible or is very precarious.

But these 'small worlds' are not in themselves apolitical.

It is possible to organize (and it is happening), even within this smallness, something like a 'second state'. We have different forms of engaging with people, organizing help, food, and sometimes – as in Berlin, where comrades occupied seven buildings – shelter, clothes, and psychological help, providing services the state cannot or does not provide.

Often these actions happen under the radar, and they might not be articulated in a political language (yet), but they are the first steps in a political direction. I hope so; these would lead into organizing a political consciousness and structures that might come in handy in the next years of crisis. I am convinced of the permanence of this social and economic crisis.

And this might be radicalized in the United States, where the state seems to be failing completely.

Milena Katsarska (5 April 2020, Plovdiv, Bulgaria)

It seems to me that the only thing keeping the situation in Bulgaria from exploding is the weather, which turned Novemberish again over the weekend, after the Parliament announced a 13 May deadline for the current state of emergency – way beyond expectations. I was wondering why Sofia University had announced its closure until 10 May as early as 25 March, many days before the currently extended deadline was announced. I suppose that might have been a reasonable projection based on taking into account the 1–6 May national holidays. I would have put the deadline there (10 May) early on, had I been asked. The logic of the current parliamentary decision escapes me, though, because one does not put a mid-week day as the end day if that's to be 'a real deadline'.

What unnerved me in this respect are two things: (1) the fringe group Volya advocated for an indefinite state of emergency, like the one put in place in Hungary,[6] and (2) Bulgaria in fact has not signed the EU-13 declaration that commits countries to maintaining the current procedural democratic arrangement, that is, to keep potential for 'dictatorship' in check. That is not good at all. The socialists were against the current prolongation; they would have preferred the end of April instead and demanded clear economic strategies. They were tentatively joined by the Movement for Rights and Freedoms, who gave a provisional 'leeway' agreement to the proposal but insisted on a transparent parliamentary discussion of economic measures/plans. In short, the move passed, but there's an indicative fissure there.

The annoying liberal elites (you know who I am talking about, those June 2013 protest guys) are rallying for the defence of Ivo Prokopiev, the non-GERB oligarch and media tycoon.[7] That is neither here nor there – again! On the surface, it is a call for the 'defense of freedom of speech', with the move to freeze all Prokopiev's assets being read as a retaliation against the publications in *Dnevnik* criticizing government actions in the current crisis.[8] Well, if one checks timelines – as one should – the court decision for this was dated 14 February after a longish due process for investigating corrupt practices. Then there was a delay of 14 days in implementing the judgement to allow for an appeal; if that one is dismissed, the next appeal can only come after the first decision has been acted upon, that is, assets frozen to the size of 200 million. This is a murky story, difficult to get to the bottom of, and it has been going through a legal procedure for quite some time. But now it has turned rhetorically into a case that 'serves the emergency situation' when executives are scrambling for such appropriated funds. In reality, though, those funds cannot really be used, simply because the legal procedure has not been concluded – but the whole issue is now being seen as designed for that purpose. That development is indicative of the rift that might blow up between the two major blocs in the country. Prokopiev has always enjoyed American backing, while over the last year, Boyko has gained considerable American backing, too. I think this unfolding drama reveals a shift in terms of 'which American spine' controls matters in Bulgaria, and it has been coming for some time.

At the same time, I am taken aback by the seeming ease and calmness with which Bulgarians are resigned to the prospect of extended measures these days. The British press speaks of 'unrest' after less than two weeks, while here – if we take into account the 'flu measures' that started around 1 March in various parts of the country and became blanket nationwide on March 8 – there's been a gradual process of limitations for a month now. I was surprised that instead of waiting for the current date, 13 April (a week before it, in fact), another month was announced; not another logical 'extension' to, say the end of April, with Easter thrown in (that's 18–19 for the Orthodox world). For this decision, the 'virus logic' doesn't really cover the matter; perhaps economic and political manoeuvres underpinning the previous observations do. It is a mess, in other words, and one that will perhaps become volatile, depending on how well the social security arrangements actually work around Easter. All those people who have been laid off will be relying now, this month, on receiving social benefits, and by and large, I think, small savings will just about last them until the end of April.

Suman Gupta (7 April 2020, Delhi, India)

Modi's call to put out the bulbs and light candles for the 5th[9] was not as successful as the go-out-and-clap of the 22nd last month. It worked out in an interesting way. A couple of days before the 5th, a chief electric engineer somewhere observed that if a sufficient number put out their lights and then switched them on again, there could be an electrical outage. Then people can carry on living with their candles. In the 24 hours leading up to the Moment, all but two of the 15 or so TV news channels we receive ran a sustained propaganda campaign to get people to bend to Modi's appeal. From an appeal, it seemed to become a directive. Reporters swarmed on TVs shrieking in great excitement about how the great Indian people were responding enthusiastically to the appeal; large quantities of little clay lamps were being manufactured; Modi's inspiration was being emulated around the world in Italy and elsewhere. On the public broadcasting site Doordarshan (which few seem to watch these days), the reporters descended to pleading, requesting viewers to *please* put out electric lights and light lamps to express their solidarity with the collective struggle. A minor BJP leader observed that those who don't put out their electric lights and light lamps are 'anti-national'. My mother's friend rang to say that in her cooperative block it was suggested that not just lights but all electrical appliances should be switched off. But then the scientific among them decided that that's not quite right: remember that chief engineer; in fact, we must put out lights but make a point of switching on as many fans and TVs as possible at the same time.

After all that, when the Moment came it turned out that the response, at least in my vicinity, was more a whimper than a bang. Some put out their lights and some didn't, some lit a few lamps and most didn't, no one flashed torches, not many people even looked out to see whether others were doing it. However, some firecrackers went off, as if it were Diwali, and the reverberations were of monumental stupidity – as if people dying in the midst of a global pandemic make for a festive occasion.

Judging by the fact that the newspapers next morning barely had a headline on it and all those TV channels were being reticent about it, I guess it wasn't a big thing anywhere in the event.

Milena Katsarska (8 April 2020, Plovdiv, India)

The Bulgarian political scene is now enjoying a farce of exchanges between the president and the prime minister and his finance minister. It's a public spat where classical quotations have a significant part. Goethe featured prominently. That started with President Radev shutting down the political charade of the moment, of the honourable representatives of the public chanting: 'Are you going to donate your salary as we MPs are doing?' The president made a statement and quoted the unimpeachably great poet to the effect that charity is a private act. He also informed all that both he and his wife had donated their March salaries many weeks earlier (along with some additional sums to retirement homes in Vidin as early as March 1) and that to him, this was not a PR stunt time. Then I heard Prime Minister Borisov himself quoting a different line from the great poet, and then his financial minster did the same (reading from a printout he had next to him on a desk). That segment of the news bulletin was better than any stand-up comedy, really.

The actually interesting developments were again to be found at the margins. An app has been developed by Bulgarian IT people and donated; it's called viru-something, must look into it. It has been downloaded by thousands of people now. It has the capacity to track users' movements, gives users information on the most 'contaminated' areas, gets your self-measured health-status updates to medical professionals, gives access and alerts to the police as to where you are and when your quarantine is lifted, and so on and so forth. I am sure much more. All in the name of you feeling 'safe' because you are monitored and volunteer 'Covid-related information'. Am very tempted to get into this for research purposes but prefer not to, to loosely quote Bartleby the Scrivener.

Then there's the one piece of news that was really somehow 'hidden' but is now opening up. The Bulgarian Bank for Development has taken a 75 million BGN loan so as to pass it on to other banks[10] – three other banks, in fact, but of course we don't know which because of all the client confidentiality fog. The Bank of Development's right to do so was questioned but quickly shut down with assurances that (1) a procedure was followed, and (2) it is within their operational remit. I didn't see any evidence provided to support either claim. Nor were the conditions of credits/loans made public in any way. God forbid someone gets a whiff of which banks need a loan so as to ensure they have coverage on their deposits from private citizens. Perhaps I should withdraw and put my meagre savings in a jar at home.

Sebastian Schuller (8 April 2020, Munich, Germany)

I have been keeping an eye on the vaccine conspiracy theorists and anti-vaccine lobby – the anti-vaxxers – amidst the Covid-19 crisis, as it reveals an interesting dynamic.

A few days after the Covid-19 measures were taken, I started to search for reactions of different conspiracy-theory scenes, starting with Germany.[11] Basically, there was nothing there, with the notable exception of prepper (survivalist) groups, which mainly debated more practical questions (how to survive the disaster they have been waiting for). However, they also discussed the possibility that this could be a coup by the globalist elite. In the first week of the lockdown, this narrative invaded esoteric conspiracy theory in the German-speaking Internet. Notable proponents radicalized the idea of Covid-19 as a cover-up and declared that dark, satanic agencies somehow used the virus (or the narrative of the pandemic) to fulfil their agenda – which should be countered by a global meditation event on the 5th of April. This narrative was mirrored by the Qanon community, which worries about 'deep state' activity against Trump, declaring at roughly the same time on different platforms that Covid-19 was but a cover-up for a Trumpian (or is it Trumpist?) intervention to bring the 'deep state' down.

So, at this point, all conspiracy theories circled around the non-existence of the virus. The virus was either perceived as a kind of hoax or, at most, as an artificial predicament, produced, perhaps on purpose, by some dark agencies.

Then this narrative began to shift slowly toward conspiracy theories connected to the anti-vaxxer movement I am particularly interested in. Basically, anti-vaxxers do not deny the existence of Covid-19 as a health condition. They may deny the existence of the virus; there are more radical anti-vaxxers, especially within the neo-Nazi and/or the anthroposophic context, who deny the existence of viruses altogether because of their belief systems. But they do not deny the impact or the disease itself. Now, the main take within this scene is that the disease is being used by Big Pharma to milk money from the state by introducing obligatory vaccination. Here, it is interesting to note that Robert F. Kennedy, Jr., a big shot in the scene, very cleverly fuels this conspiracy theory by posting nice little stories on his *Children's Health Defense* website of how Vitamin D could save us all from Covid-19, implying between the lines that all the costly measures to save patients are not necessary but serve the profit interest of Big Pharma.[12] As it happens, Robert is a very mild conspiracy theorist. The hegemonic tendency within the anti-vaxxer community is to assume that Covid-19 is related to 5G antennas. This is a topic already present for some time within this scene (Robert put up an article on this on the same website)[13] which is taking off now. An air of conspiracy around 5G networks has been firmly fostered by various states (starting with the United States, Australia, and United Kingdom from 2019), which banned the use of Chinese equipment produced by Huawei in their 5G networks on the grounds that these are being designed by the Chinese government for espionage. The racist anti-Chinese current which has followed the course of the Covid-19 contagion throughout found an unexpected sideline in anti-vaxxer circles.

There are two strains to this. The assumption is either that 5G has negative effects on the immune system, which creates the condition for Covid-19 to infect the body, or that 5G is the direct cause of the disease itself (in these extremities of lunacy, the second goes further). In any case, the narrative goes that the disease was effected by electromagnetic radiation and is now being used by Big Pharma and the state to follow through with dark, profit-driven plans. For that reason, some groups resolved on burning down 5G antennas (these strains and some militant actions of these groups are usefully summed up in an article by article by Kiera Butler).[14] Taking off by the beginning of April, these medical anti-vaxxer conspiracy theories are slowly replacing the more 'political' and esoteric conspiracy theories and are now gaining ground. It is noteworthy that they originate almost exclusively in the Anglosphere but are now received by German conspiracy theory forums. Some have started to adjust to this new narrative, thus ultimately accepting the existence of the disease.

We see two points of interest here.

First, my feeling (I haven't done enough research to be categorical) is that this is a rather typical movement within the Western conspiracy scene, which goes as follows. A given event happens. Immediately after the event, only a few conspiracy theories are produced, most of them rather wild and unconnected. Then, some weeks into the event, when a plethora of contradictory and heteroform texts have already emerged, finally a master conspiracy theory appears, usually in the Anglosphere. This allows for the organization of a fragile unity within the conspiracy theory chaos. The central points of this master conspiracy theory are slowly integrated within the diverse texts and sometimes modified. Only a very few conspiracy theory texts obdurately separate themselves from that master conspiracy theory and do not relate to it.

Second, it is at least a curious coincidence that this trajectory mirrors the inner movement of the far right in the United States. In January and most of February, far-right commentators decried Covid-19 as a hoax put out by Democrats . . . echoed by Trump himself. As the contagion hit the United States, they made a U-turn and called for national measures and so on. These turns are somehow mirrored by the international conspiracy theory scene, especially the anti-vaxxer movement. This suggests that the scene is dependent on crucial rightwing US commentators and thinkers, though that might not be apparent from the European perspective.

Suman Gupta (8 April 2020, Delhi, India)

Sebastian – some thoughts follow on your interesting observations on the anti-vaxxer scene.

1   The kind of conspiracy theory I know you are interested in – anti-vaxxer, flat-earthers, prepper, ET, Holocaust denial, and so on – seems to be expressive of a particular sort of alienated consciousness. On the one hand, it appears to be alienated from mainstream consensus grounded on reason and evidence: the more firmly grounded, the more strongly is the refusal expressed from the alienated position. Naturally, scientific and historical consensus is most obviously grounded in reason and evidence, and taking the opposite position to those seems the obvious option for this kind of alienation. On the other hand, this extreme alienation is manifested in a desire for something of that which it refutes – a new consensus based on a simulation of the same kind of grounding, so that such conspiracy theories present tortuous reasonings and

scattergun selective information and misinformation to justify themselves and pull together as in-groups. Both the refusal and the desire are expressive of this kind of alienated consciousness.

2   While the alienation entails a refusal of mainstream consensus based on reason and evidence while desiring something akin to it, there are, increasingly, mainstream elements which underpin this sort of alienation – or, rather, a mainstream environment which *produces* it. (1) Commodity marketing constantly gives the impression that each consumer has a right to choose a lifestyle and determine how the world should be according to their desires. (2) A pervasive management and consultancy culture suggests that any product, including worldviews, can be instilled by following sustained publicity and manipulation strategies irrespective of empirical realities. (3) Religious institutions have ever trodden cautiously around or directly rejected scientific or historical evidence and reasoning. (4) Political opportunists on the right have increasingly and successfully made breaking such consensus their credo.

3   The digital environment accentuates those mainstream elements which tacitly encourage the kind of conspiracy-theory alienation in question. This environment enables: withdrawal from communal or collective interactions where those evidence-and-reason-based consensuses are functional; access to a field of communications where targeting according to established attitudes is a pervasive practice; availability of equipment to search and locate others of similar disposition, however widely dispersed; the ability to rapidly disperse misinformation on the back of affective qualities (sensational, outrageous, hyperbolic, etc.). These are all features which could bolster this kind of conspiracy-theory alienation.

4   The condition of institutionalized global social isolation brings all these elements into a totality – this might be, I am thinking, the ideal condition for the universalization of conspiracy theories. It might lead to a master conspiracy theory building upon the direction you point to, a consolidation which brings together various strands and misdirections into a kind of whole.

I have not expressed the last point as clearly as I would like to – but there's a niggle somewhere in there to sharpen.

Notes

1 'Jeremy Corbyn's last prime minister's questions', *UK Parliament*, 25 March 2020, www.youtube.com/watch?v=-dABvHq-wkY (accessed 30 May 2020).
2 'PM Modi's video message on COVID-19', *Rajya Sabha TV*, 3 April 2020, www.youtube.com/watch?v=W5L-1kfLJg (accessed 30 May 2020).
3 Ernesto Londoño, Manuela Andreoni and Letícia Casado, 'Bolsonaro, isolated and defiant, dismisses coronavirus threat to Brazil', *New York Times*, 1 April 2020, www.nytimes.com/2020/04/01/world/americas/brazil-bolsonaro-coronavirus.html (accessed 30 May 2020).
4 Tom Phillips, 'Bolsonaro threatens to sack health minister over coronavirus criticism', *Guardian*, 29 March 2020, www.theguardian.com/world/2020/mar/29/

bolsonaro-warns-health-minister-covid-19; Gabriel Stargardter and Lisandra Para-guassu, 'One Brazilian minister shines as coronavirus clobbers Bolsonaro', *Reuters*, 1 April 2020, https://in.reuters.com/article/health-coronavirus-brazil-minister-newsm/ one-brazilian-minister-shines-as-coronavirus-clobbers-bolsonaro-idINKBN21J69I; Thais Arbex and Renata Mariz, 'Bolsonaro se irritou com suposta 'arrogância' de Man-detta', *O Globo*, 3 April 2020, https://oglobo.globo.com/brasil/bolsonaro-se-irritou-com-suposta-arrogancia-de-mandetta-24348521 (accessed 30 May 2020).

5 Gustavo Ribeiro, 'Poll: Brazilians reject Bolsonaro's coronavirus approach', *Brazilian Report*, 3 April 2020, https://brazilian.report/coronavirus-brazil-live-blog/2020/04/03/ poll-brazilians-reject-bolsonaro-coronavirus-approach/ (accessed 30 May 2020).

6 'Депутатите в спор за срока на извънредното положение – до 30 април или до 13 май', *Investor.bg*, 13 April 2020, www.investor.bg/ikonomika-i-politika/332/a/depu-tatite-v-spor-za-sroka-na-izvynrednoto-polojenie-do-30-april-ili-do-13-mai-301810/ (accessed 30 May 2020).

7 The case of corruption against Ivo Prokpiev mentioned here is of longer standing, for the context see: 'Oligarch Prokopiev with a new plot to get out of debt', *Europost*, 14 October 2019, https://europost.eu/en/a/view/oligarch-prokopiev-with-a-new-plot-to-get-out-of-debt-26461. On news of the order to seize his property, which this inter-vention responds to, see: Krasen Nikolov, 'Иво Прокопиев: Щабът за политическа репресия е активен по време на кризат', *mediapool.bg*, 31 March 2020, www.medi apool.bg/ivo-prokopiev-shtabat-za-politicheska-represiya-e-aktiven-po-vreme-na-krizata-news305513.html; 'Запорираха още акции и имущество на Иво Прокопиев', *news.bg*, 31 March 2020 (accessed 30 May 2020).

8 Prokopiev is owner of newspapers *Kapital* and *Dnevnik*. For a critical article on his hold on Bulgarian media, see: 'Prokopiev holds mainstream media through bTV, Dnevnik and Capital', *Europost*, 3 February 2020, https://europost.eu/en/a/view/prokopiev-holds-mainstream-media-through-b-tv-dnevnik-and-capital-27220 (accessed 30 May 2020).

9 Ostensibly as a gesture of solidarity of Indian citizens in the fight against Covid-19, 'PM Modi's video message on COVID-19', *Rajya Sabha TV*, 3 April 2020, www.youtube. com/watch?v=W5L-1kfLJg (accessed 30 May 2020).

10 The loan was approved on 26 March 2020. See: 'Банката за развитие отпусна 75 млн. лв. на фирма почти без дейност', *Dnevnik*, 6 April 2020, www.dnevnik. bg/biznes/2020/04/06/4051178_bankata_za_razvitie_otpusna_75_mln_lv_na_ firma_pochti/; 'Нов голям съмнителен кредит на ББР: 75 млн. лв. за свързана със "С. Г. груп" компания', *Kapital,* 6 April 2020, www.capital.bg/biznes/ finansi/2020/04/06/4050919_nov_goliam_sumnitelen_kredit_na_bbr_75_mln_lv_ za/. It led to Borisov firing the director of the BBD, Stoyan Mavrodiev, and some board members due to the public outcry and oppositional political backlash that followed, in a matter of 24 hours or so, as reported here: 'Борисов разпореди Мавродиев да бъде освободен като директор на ББР', *Investor.bg*, 8 April 2020, www.investor.bg/biudjet-i-finansi/333/a/borisov-razporedi-mavrodiev-da-byde-osvoboden-kato-direktor-na-bbr-302046/ (accessed 30 May 2020).

11 Shortly after this, a Cornell University 'Alliance for Science' blog was written that gave a useful list of Covid-19 conspiracy theories: Mark Lynas, 'COVID: Top 10 current conspiracy theories', *Cornell Alliance for Science*, 20 April 2020, https://allianceforsci-ence.cornell.edu/blog/2020/04/covid-top-10-current-conspiracy-theories/ (accessed 30 May 2020). There have been numerous news features, documentaries, blogs, videos, and so on earlier and since addressing conspiracy theories around the pandemic. These understood the space in terms of what such theories assert – their content – rather than in terms of the social organization of the space – what groups exist through what chan-nels and in what relation. The names given to or assumed by such groups or bringing together like-minded groups (such as 'prepper', 'anti-vaxxer', 'Qanon'), and the various appellations that crisscross across them, breaking them into subgroups or linking them, are largely in the zone of a kind of insider knowledge – either through being part of such a scene or by being a watcher of such scenes.

12 Katie Weisman and the CHD Team, 'COVID-19 and Vitamin D: Could we be missing something simple?' *Children's Health Defence*, 7 April 2020, https://childrenshealth defense.org/news/covid-19-and-vitamin-d-could-we-be-missing-something-simple/ (accessed 30 May 2020).

13 A. Naran, et al., 'Electromagnetic radiation due to cellular, Wi-Fi and Bluetooth technologies: How safe are we?' *Children's Health Defence*, 7 April 2020, https:// childrenshealthdefense.org/child-health-topics/known-culprit/electromagnetic/ electromagnetic-radiation-due-to-cellular-wi-fi-and-bluetooth-technologies-how-safe-are-we/ (accessed 30 May 2020).

14 Kiera Butler, '"A fake pandemic": Anti-vaxxers are spreading coronavirus conspiracy theories', *Mother Jones*, 24 March 2020, www.motherjones.com/politics/2020/03/a-fake-pandemic-antivaxxers-are-spreading-coronavirus-conspiracy-theories/ (accessed 30 May 2020).

5

OF PROTESTS

Summary: *The Covid-19 lockdowns ended some prolonged and very determined protests in various parts of the world. This chapter begins by taking note of these and wonders what the prospects for protests might be under lockdown – given that the ways in which lockdowns are enacted may themselves be unjust. Later in the chapter, the possible means of online protests are examined, with ambiguous conclusions. Woven amidst these preoccupations, developments on some of the political fronts of lockdown are described, as is the uneventful flow of everyday life in seclusion.*

Suman Gupta (9 April 2020, Delhi, India)

The Citizenship (Amendment) Act (CAA) 2019 makes it legal for the Indian state to grant refugee status to Hindus, Sikhs, Buddhists, Jains, Parsis, and Christians who have suffered and escaped religious persecution in Pakistan, Bangladesh, and Afghanistan. Muslims were pointedly left out, as were Ahmadiyyas and non-believers and rationalists (with or without Muslim names), who often fall foul of religious laws and are persecuted by religious organizations. The legislation was concerned only with the three neighbouring Muslim-dominated countries and didn't seem troubled about other neighbouring countries (China, Myanmar, Sri Lanka, Nepal, Bhutan). Most significantly, this is legislation which makes religion explicitly the grounds for inclusion in or exclusion from governmental policy and implicitly makes religious affiliation a norm for Indian citizenship – against constitutional guarantees. Combined with other current government proposals, ostensibly to combat illegal immigration (such as that of a National Register of Citizens or NCR), a dangerous drift towards ethnic cleansing could be suspected.

On 24 March 2020, two days after the Covid-19 lockdown was announced across India, the most remarkable peaceful protest action since Independence ended, with police removing the remaining protesters. Since around mid-December 2019, a street was occupied in Shaheen Bagh in Delhi to protest against the passing of CAA in both houses of Parliament. Around the same time, a video clip of the brutal police action in Jamia Millia University against student protesters engaging the same issue (and also possibly just random students in that university) was widely circulated in the international media: police were recorded entering the university library and beating up students.[1] The Shaheen Bagh protest was organized predominantly by Muslim women in the area. Various student and activist groups joined them. The demand to repeal CAA gathered the status of a wider opposition against BJP's Hindu nationalist ideology and offered a different vision of the nation. Various Supreme Court petitions and police pressure to remove it proved unsuccessful.[2] Lumpen youth from the provinces travelled to Delhi with firearms to shoot at the protesters twice, to no avail.[3] The Covid-19 lockdown in Delhi from 23 March offered an unassailable reason to shut the protest and remove/detain the protesters. The protesters had tried to abide by the Covid-19 restrictions up to then, sitting at the requisite distance from each other and wearing face masks and gloves but refusing to remove the occupation.

In early 2020, sustained mass and street protests were being reported in the mainstream media in Hong Kong, Iraq, Iran, Lebanon, Canada, Mexico, Chile, Brazil, Columbia, France, Italy, Poland, Algeria, Liberia . . . to name a few. Most were variously against anti-austerity policies, authoritarian policies, and gender violence. Widely dispersed protest actions concerning climate change and environmental depredation were constantly in the news. These protest movements struggled vainly against the overwhelming call for Covid-19 social distancing restrictions as the virus spread, before fizzing out and disappearing – if not in spirit, in notable presence on the streets and squares and in the media.

This raises some pressing questions. Does the seeming suspension of politics under lockdown necessarily mean the automatic suspension of *all* protest? Going by the principle that all social considerations have been reorganized around the imperative centrality of Covid-19 social distancing, many of the issues that have aroused active disquiet so far (austerity, authoritarianism, xenophobia, migration, religious/class/caste/race/gender/sexuality conflicts, climate change) have either gone on the back burner or been deferred for an indefinite return to business as usual which may never be quite as usual even if the contagion subsides.

But then, the very management of Covid-19 by the state apparatuses of different governments could give plenty of cause for disquiet and dissent. This is not just a matter of not acting upon restrictions. How that implementation is messaged and managed offers wide scope for governmental/media/corporate malfeasance. For instance, in various ways, testing and support for the infected could be tacitly limited to some sectors of a population rather than others; the lockdown could be implemented so as to exploit/oppress the marginalized or clamp down on rights/activist organizations; various agencies may engage in extortionate practices on an anxious population; government agents may conduct xenophobic and implicitly genocidal propaganda on the back of Covid-19. . . . If the managers of the lockdown are also the agents of malfeasance *enabled by the lockdown*, what's the recourse? How should effective protest be expressed – within the parameters of social distancing?

[Have to make a note of this: as I am writing this, in a warm late afternoon in an apartment of a middle-class East Delhi cooperative block, in the next cooperative block – appropriately called Prayer Apartments – a Hindu religious meeting is proceeding in full swing. Bhajans are being sung, prayers chanted, cries of 'Jai Shri Ram' . . . some 25 or 30 people are on the lawn, no masks, not particularly distant from each other. They aren't hiding, either, since the proceedings are being blasted out on loudspeakers. They have been at it almost all day, and the front road is remarkably free of police today. What social distancing? Whither lockdown? No one around seems bothered; my neighbours are suitably isolated and seemingly deaf – I have a good view of the devout gathering from my window . . .]

Of course, responsible pillars of society would say that this is no time for protests about anything – complaints should be lodged though the proper channels to the appropriate authorities, and proceedings will be instituted after the crisis is managed or when an opportunity arises for conducting a disinterested investigation. This sort of response doesn't inspire confidence even when there isn't a state of emergency and social distancing isn't the rule of the day – if they did, protests wouldn't ever need to happen. Even under what's regarded as normal circumstances, the proper channels (with the ombudsmen, the police, the investigators, judicial functionaries) often seem to be designed to undertake the defence of the state or corporate agency accused of wrongdoing as its default position – Kafka's novel *The Trial* could be regarded as a philosophical essay on this default position. In a state of emergency and lockdown, even that default position seems in abeyance. Distraction from addressing complaints because of a raging pandemic is an easy excuse. Moreover, a certain impatience on the part of the pillars of society and the appropriate authorities may be expected. There can't be a more dangerous moment to be seen as protesting. The state with emergency powers, a people on edge and frazzled, and a feverish environment are not amenable to protest, however polite and peaceful that protest might be. To protest in these circumstances is to court punitive suppression, more precipitate than the generally impatient and brutish ways in which protests are usually dealt with by the state. And yet the issue that spurs dissent and protest may well be at the heart of the health crisis itself, a critical moment of self-preservation, not unlike the Shaheen Bagh protests until 24 March 2020.

There is a direct incompatibility between conventional strategies of social protest and an instituted condition of social distancing. Most expressions of protest involve collective presence, the appearance of the protesting crowd: the march, the rally, the demonstration, filling the town square or gathering before the parliament, meeting at the picket line or the barricade . . . or, for that matter, turning riotous, storming the Bastille or the Winter Palace. At the core of the protesting crowd, the most effective and historically charted form of social protest is the combination of the threat of force and the legitimacy of collective demand. Fear of the crowd could well be the lynchpin of political theory and practice under every sort of regime since the Roman Republic. From their inception, formally democratic and liberal capitalist regimes have obsessively tried to formulate the character and mind of the crowd – ever on the verge of turning uncontrollable or revolutionary – so as to be able to control it. From Gustave Le Bon's (1869) diatribes against the crowd-mind where conscious constraints drop away, to Elias Canetti's (1960) politically charged observations on the shapes and movements of crowds, to Philip Zimbardo's (1969) scientific-sounding concepts of the deindividuated person in the crowd/group in the later 20th century,[4] and then on to the development of crowd surveillance and crowd management specialisms . . . crowding renders protest effective because it suggests a dangerous *force*. Even if it is in fact quite a peaceable and disciplined crowd that gathers to object to, say, something like the CAA, its appearance suggests a latent and simmering threat, a potential for exerting force. At the same time, the protesting crowd seemingly claims democratic legitimacy. It now frequently claims and is accepted as representing the will of the demos – an alternative to the managed and controlled (and variously riggable) form of general elections/referendums as representing the will of the people. Every anti-war, anti-austerity, anti-corruption, and so on protesting collective action has made this claim and effectively. The idea of the really large crowd (the number is the key, always contested between police and organizers of protests) as having democratic legitimacy has settled as democratic norms have garnered a powerful, if often unconsidered, normative consensus. The protesting crowd is a threatening force, and the protesting crowd represents the demos – between these concepts, we have the concretization of the most powerful form of social protest or dissent.

Social distancing is the absolute annulment of that kind of threat and that kind of claim to legitimacy. It is at the opposite pole of sociality where protest as crowding, as collective presence, is possible. If social distancing obtains scientific and popular consensus and becomes an institutionalized social condition, as it does while the Covid-19 pandemic ravages (hopefully not beyond that) – then *what forms of effective social protest remain which have a similar force and a similar sense of democratic legitimacy?*

There's a question . . . [to be continued some time]

Milena Katsarska (9 April 2020, Plovdiv, Bulgaria)

I agree with these observations on protest in Covid-19 times. That is an important consideration, not only theoretically what happens to protest in these times but also very practically, in view of the immediate cease-and-desist of many protests – not only in India but also in all those other locations mentioned. If nothing could stop Hong Kong protesters for a year, Covid-19 or, to be precise, the state's declared measures for the all-consuming objective of preserving human life, definitely and definitively did. This could very well be the newly discovered mechanism that states can enjoy and deploy. Then the question is that which is posed at the end.

There are all sorts of other questions that come to mind as well. In the middle ground between, on the one hand, ideas of democracy and legitimacy and, on the other hand, the practicality of gathering as a protesting crowd, the immediate situation limits realistic options severely. In any case, at present, protests can be contemplated if addressed (1) against state-imposed measures because of Covid-19 or (2) a social issue that has surfaced against the background of Covid-19 measures. With regard to (2), that could be issues to do with poverty, 'casual employment', unemployment, homelessness, and so on. These are obviously social issues with or without Covid-19. However, against the background of lockdowns, it becomes possible for state and corporate and international agencies to explain them away as peculiarly down to Covid-19. Where it might have been apparent that those issues were consequent on sustained government policies across time, now they are apt to seem conditional to Covid-19, exacerbated because of that, visible because of that, under discussion because of that, and so on. And instead of interrogating state ideologies and policies, such issues become subject to sympathetic calls for charitable moves, occasional donations and concessions, and so on, which effectively depoliticize them.

An example of such an issue, for instance, is that of domestic violence. This is interestingly one of the first issues of long standing that has acquired a special position amidst the Covid-19 lockdowns – so far, much more so than homelessness or poverty. But that is just as a matter of 'let's talk more about it and talk about it now' and solve it quickly so that it becomes a non-issue before that overwhelming issue – not in the spirit of protests.

Incidentally, on a different note: there's a curious electronic centralization of data going on in universities here. It involves collecting data about the physical presence of lecturers in classrooms and submitting that to a central platform. This is an attempt to get to the reality of *physical* teaching and *physical* learning presence, not the usual symbolic double-weighting of lectures compared to seminars, or the symbolic reductions of weightings for smaller groups that have usually occupied our accountants. Now there is a gathering of data on bodies in real time in university classrooms. I daresay this data-gathering exercise was planned before the lockdown; it isn't easy to have such a platform in place so quickly. Anyway, the platform has to be fed this data by universities, which will then be centrally processed. The Central Commission for Academic whatever declares this is for the purposes of determining university ratings. Sure, that's right, but maybe that's not even the half of it. It is only as of yesterday that the depth of detail required emerged and our university higher-ups got slightly worried. It would be a headache to collect, but one might think that once done, it's done. But that is not the case. The case is that the required data is directly related, at one end, to salary calculations in any unit's budget and, at the other end, to rating the state subsidy to any unit's budget again. The relationship between physical presence and economy in the university classroom is beginning to be estimated more closely than ever, just as the Covid-19 lockdowns have taken those bodies away from those classrooms.

John Seed (10 April 2020, London, United Kingdom)

As far as I can see, which isn't far, everything around is calm and very quiet. Few people and fewer cars pass by. I went for a stroll the other day, and it was eerily quiet. The occasional person you spot a hundred yards ahead slinks away nervously as if you have bubonic plague. I gather it's pretty much the same everywhere. All shops are shut except supermarkets and pharmacies, so city centres are empty. You can hear noisy kids playing in their gardens. But parks are now mostly shut, as, of course, are cinemas, theatres, restaurants, everywhere people socialize.

Most people seem to be stoics and accept that they are confined to their homes and gardens and can't see family or friends, so let's make the best of it. I gather incidents of domestic violence have increased significantly – as they do during the Christmas break. Alcohol sales have increased. A report on the BBC last night said that a minority of people – was it around 20% – are really struggling with anxiety and sleeplessness. But most people seem to be making the best of things.[5] Every Thursday night at 20:00 throughout the United Kingdom, people go onto the street and cheer and blow horns and bang pots for a couple of minutes of celebration of the work of the NHS. Outside here last night, hundreds of people were outside making noise.

But a lot of those people know their future is uncertain in terms of jobs. The 14% drop in economic activity is fairly catastrophic and makes the 2008 crash look like a minor blip.[6]

As for myself, my life is 90% the same as it was before. But I feel unsettled and struggle to concentrate. It's like I am waiting for something, but I am not sure what. I haven't seen anybody but C for 24 days, which reminds me that she hasn't seen anybody but me – which evens things out. She potters in the garden, reads one of her women novelists or watches one of her Jane Austen box sets; I lie on the bed and read and scribble notes and trawl YouTube and listen to music – and do 4–5 miles on my exercise bike while watching all 74 episodes of *Death in Paradise*. I try to cook something interesting every day. I eat well and sleep well. The days slip by quickly. But I suppose we are all aware that out of sight, every hospital is packed with the sick and the dying in a tidal wave of suffering that has no end in sight yet.

Fabio Akcelrud Durão (11 April 2020, São Carlos, São Paulo State, Brazil)

Things are happening so fast that it is impossible to think about them properly. All we can do is try to guess and run the risk of being proven wrong in less than a week. Just a couple of months ago, I was considering a Bolsonaro self-coup feasible;[7] then I started to believe that he was about to fall. Four days ago, the polls gave him a solid 33% approval rate after he gave a seemingly conciliatory address on TV despite ongoing conflict with the health minister Mandetta[8] – but then we have to wait for the bodies to start appearing because of the virus.

Now I hear a rumour (the cherry on the ice cream) that there is a legal request to make former President Lula da Silva's Workers' Party (PT) illegal,[9] which would devastate the Left for the next elections and years to come. So, in view of all this, all I can do during the quarantine is to get some popcorn and watch whatever (and despair, of course . . .). It's so hard to concentrate with all this instability. Every night I pray to Jesus for a normal, standard neoliberal right-wing president and judiciary.

Milena Katsarska (11 April 2020, Plovdiv, Bulgaria)

Over my morning coffee, I tuned into the TV segment where there was a good interview with the former Finance Minister Milen Velchev[10] (he was some top manager in Merrill Lynch, a job he left so as to join the government of Simeon). I think he's been living primarily in London again because I had coincidentally been on two flights from London to Sofia with his family, but now he's here. From a financial point of view, he was realistically brutal in, for instance, citing current electricity consumption in the American context, which is already worse than in 2008 as an indicator of a deeper economic dive now. Being firmly of a neoliberal disposition insofar as I can see (it was under his leadership, after all, that the last two commerce banks were privatized in Bulgaria), he stated that the 10 billion credit/ debt that Bulgaria is contemplating should not even be a matter of parliamentary debate/approval; it should simply be immediately done. The favourable conditions for this are on the table now and might not be there in a short while. Per capita financial eases are unnecessary because Bulgaria's social system offers enough of a safety net (for now). And ultimately (those savings!) there is a 'significant mass' of people in Bulgaria who have savings, and they will see those savings vanish, but that will tide them over, and so on and so forth.

As predicted, the political rifts between institutions in Bulgaria are deepening, most notably between the government and the presidency, but also within different political parties in parliament. In society there are also signs of pushes for divisions in all sorts of ways. Those could be symbolic along the lines of, say, 'urban young-sters are not quite following the rules' (and are jeopardizing everybody's health, especially those following them) but also of a more serious nature as questions like this begin to emerge, 'Why don't they (executives/establishment) cordon off certain neighbourhoods?' That implies compact ethnic neighbourhoods or pro-vincial working-class 'riff raff' in Sofia block residential areas. There are idiotic but serious calls to designate the Orthodox clergy as an 'at risk frontline group' so that the group gets priority testing (like doctors, police, firefighters, etc.). That's so that Bulgarians can cluster in a church, believe it or not. Of all places, out of all the reasons in the world. The latter calls were nicely shut down by our main pro-tagonist the General earlier today, but I don't think it will be up to him ultimately. Then there are pushes for further exceptions to the state of exception that are to do with finances, benefits, employment, and so on. One could say that the so-called solidarity in the face of a crisis or under humanitarian concerns is anything but solidarity if it begins to crack so easily along class, ethnic, religious, and other lines.

Suman Gupta (11 April 2020, Delhi, India)

[. . . carrying on about protests and Covid lockdowns . . .]

If physical gatherings – any kind of crowding – to protest become impossible, then the obvious way for protest to go would be into the digital space. Just as under Covid-19 lockdowns, a significant part of white-collar, service-sector, middle-class work has moved online, all protests could seek to move online, too. Let me consider what the prospects are.

There are two general issues to bear in mind.

1   The most significant protests often come from below, from lower-income groups and variously marginalized populations – for obvious reasons. These are precisely the people who are least likely to capitalize effectively on the resources of digital environments. Digital divides are very far from bridged, even where uptake of digital resources is seemingly high. There are two levels of divide to do with two dimensions of access.

   •   First, there is raw access – simply to be able to enter and function in this environment. This is a matter of what sort of gadget one has, what sorts of broadband speeds are available, what the costs of internet services are, and so on. In countries with large poor populations, raw access is far from universal. In India, for instance, internet access was very optimistically estimated at 34% in 2017, and by 2021, this is expected to become around 50% – going with that, the 50% who still won't have any kind of access are probably dominated by the poor.

   •   Second, even after raw access, there are levels of access from basic to high functionality and according to the ability to afford services. That range depends upon level of education, technical expertise, amount of time spent on developing experience, income, and so on – which are all areas in which lower-income and marginalized persons are disadvantaged even if they did have reasonable raw access. Given these disadvantages of access, lower-income and marginalized groups with a grievance to protest about are likely to have less autonomy than otherwise. They would have to depend to some extent upon sympathetic middle-class tech-savvy activists to champion their cause and pronounce in their name. More importantly, they would have to depend upon largely private digital service providers who enable suitable access for a cost or public providers which offer subsidized access but are themselves agencies of the state security apparatus – that is, depend upon parties who are likely causes of grievances.

2   The digital environment, insofar as publicly acknowledged, is comprehensively policed and recorded, with very few (not very effective) laws governing the regulation of such policing and recording. A collective protest would usually seek a public arena, whether that's a town square in a city or a *bona fide* network in digital space. The *bona fide* network, however, allows for maximum

exposure with minimum regulatory protection. Protesters are vulnerable to various kinds of covert retaliatory or suppressive methods in digital space which would be considered illegal and certainly unethical in real space. Of course, there are low-visibility and intractable parts of the digital environment – these pertain to protests as the back alley to the high street. So, the *modus operandi* of protests in digital space need to be devoted as much to drawing attention as to evading suppression and retaliation.

With these general points in mind, let me pause upon some of the ways in which protests relate to digital space.

1   The most-discussed aspect of digital capacities in protests has been as tools for the organization and coordination of crowd protests, enhancing their threat of force and the sense of democratic legitimacy. This is therefore not relevant to the situation in question here, that is, the possibilities of protest under conditions of lockdown, like the ongoing Covid-19 one, in pure digital space. Nevertheless, this prolific area of commentary has a few points of interest.

- Especially from the so-called series of 'Arab Spring' uprisings, late 2010 onwards, to the Hong Kong protests which were effectively overcome by the Covid-19 outbreak, the use of social networking tools by organizers of and participants in mass demonstrations has featured regularly in news media and academic publications. Initially, the role of Twitter and Facebook was especially noted – some significant protest movements came to be labelled 'Twitter revolutions' – and numerous other apps and providers have been called upon since. Though social networking tools were no more than tools, there has been a tendency to attribute a sort of autonomous impetus to them (as in the phrase 'Twitter revolutions'), often so as to obfuscate the strategic roles of ideologues and organizing agencies. To some extent, this shows how seamlessly the commercial interests of social-network providers (digital entrepreneurs) co-opt the energies of large-scale protests. Even in the interstitial part played by digital tools in crowd protests, at some level, the protests themselves turn into ambient advertising for the entrepreneurs.
- On a different note, just as digital tools have facilitated crowd protests, digital tools have also been honed to work against crowd protests: sophisticated face-recognition surveillance systems have been deployed and protesters prosecuted later or held on record; crowd modelling is used to physically manage protests; social networks are also activated to conduct propaganda against protests and initiate counter-protests. From the protesters' point of view, the play of evasion and tracking, coordination and flexibility, disruption and order, and so on that digital tools bring to crowd protests are well worth studying . . . and may have a bearing on how protests in the pure digital space work.

2   Insofar as pure digital space is in question, the more obvious strategies of protest action have to do with online campaigning. The easiest to tap into are petition and campaign web services, which have acquired a profile for channelling protest petitions of various sorts which could get significant visibility – mainly by garnering support in the form of signatories. The two that come to my mind immediately are change.org and Avaaz. It would appear that under Covid-19 lockdowns, their uptake has increased. Alexa.com maintains a ranking of global internet engagement for digital platforms: on 6 February 2020, change.org was ranked 3,410 and Avaaz 17,323; by 6 April 2020, change.org improved its ranking to 2,307 and Avaaz to 10,921. This has, then, been a period of growing online petitions, mostly to do with Covid-19, from local and issue specific to national and international and broad based. There are several features to note here re: protests.

   • First, they host an enormous variety of petitions, and there isn't a coherent ideological line for protests to align with. But then, that has increasingly been the nature of anti-war, anti-authoritarian, and anti-austerity crowd protests, encouraging diverse participation around an issue of the moment.
   • Second, as collective protest, a campaign's success is measured purely by the number of supporters: usually signatures in support. These numbers can in principle hit scales which dwarf most large crowd demonstrations. But even with impressive numbers, these have a miniscule effect compared to crowd demonstrations. Everyone knows that it takes a minute or so to sign an online petition and real effort and commitment for a crowd to get together. The crowd inevitably has at least a latent potential of force, while a petition is more like a plea which is made as soon as the signature is added. A petition gives an easy choice to the petitioned – to refuse. One of the biggest recent petitions that comes to mind was against Brexit in the United Kingdom in March 2019, with some 6 million signatories; it was simply put aside after a routine parliamentary debate.[11]
   • Third, the provider of the platform for petitions may well be out of synch with the intent of the protest petition. It is widely noted, for instance, that change.org is a profit-making venture (and should be using the .com rather than .org field), though promoting itself as a non-profit social enterprise. Avaaz is a non-profit platform.[12] The Brexit petition mentioned previously was through a platform provided by the UK Parliament which automatically raises issues which are supported by more than 10,000 signatures in Parliament.[13] This facility could be regarded as designed to raise awareness in Parliament or to manage and dilute discontent by a bureaucratic procedure.
   • Fourth, usually, working against every issue-based protest petition and campaign, there exist stable, professional, and extremely well-funded campaigning technostructures owned by the governments and corporations against which protests are often directed. These are backed by tried-and-tested propaganda strategies, existing data on online audiences,

sophisticated message-targeting capabilities, and publicists who devote all their time to making these work. If protests are to work against or to emulate such abilities, protest networks may need to set up their own technostructure and not depend upon digital service providers.

3   Hacktivism offers another and rather more controversial recourse for protesters. Basically, this involves the exploitation of system lapses within or use of customized digital tools against the systems offered (openly or by subscription) by platform and service providers. That is done either with a view to directly disrupting the operations of some agency (a hack) which the protests are directed against *as an act of protest* or revealing otherwise concealed information about such an agency (a leak) so as *to arouse protest and dissent*. There are several points to take into account here.

- First, hacktivism is mainly done by a tech-savvy constituency which is proportionally so small and, in many ways, removed from political life and contact with different strata of society that it is very unlikely to have the kind of democratic legitimacy that a large crowd or well-supported petition has. Given the paucity in appeal to numbers, the main recourse hacktivists have is to garner support by clearly articulated and evidenced argument. This is rarely found in hacktivist circles, in my experience.
- Second, the digital space for hacktivism tends to be the most coercively legislated against – it is, simply, criminalized wholesale (roughly in line with anti-terrorist or anti-fraud legislation). Operational disruption and revelation of sensitive information are precisely the kinds of things that state and commercial agencies fear most, and both gigantic investments in security systems and the most punitive retributions for perpetration of legal offences are in place. This is one of the trickiest areas for protest action, and in public perception, the line between legitimate protest and potential anti-social activity may seem blurred in this area.
- Third, it is nevertheless interesting that some of the resources that could be used for this area of protest activity (such as Tor software, blockchain technology, certain kinds of encryption and decoding systems) are not in themselves illegal. That's because they are used by state and corporate agencies for their own security and covert operations. To some degree, we may say that there's an umbilical relationship between the technological resources which sustain powerful alignments and those that can be used against them by dissenting alignments.

Milena Katsarska (11 April 2020, Plovdiv, Bulgaria)

Hmm, stuff regarding technology and protest is tricky. Whichever scenario I play out in my head, some sort of physical activity/movement is called for.

So, I started revolving imaginary scenarios that involve a lockdown situation, and those all call for a bit of Machiavellian cunning in medieval hues. Let's say the current establishment worry is: (1) keeping populations in place (we will leave the 'apart' aspect aside for the moment) and possibly (2) being aware where the population is, what the population is doing, taking stock of the population. An effective sign of protest might then be to make it difficult for an establishment to ascertain where the population is, what it is doing, and so on. That involves considerable degrees of coordinated switching off, I would say, and a wilful removal of oneself from detectable channels of presence – from social media, shopping sites, phones, and so on. Also, another sort of switching off could be, say, not using lights/electricity, TV, and a number of other appliances/gadgets that project external signs that a population is there (at home) doing predictable things. The population might still remain there, that is, where they are, but the idea is that there will be next to nothing (short of a physical entering into a residence) to ascertain the presence or absence of said population where it is 'supposed to be'. A bit of a Schrödinger's population in this imaginary scenario, and if that Schrödinger's cohort reaches a critical mass, then I bet the uncertainty principle in action will drive establishments/managers mad.

In full awareness, no such ideal situations are quite possible; I am simply letting my fantasy roam on this sunny and quite warm Saturday afternoon.

Maitrayee Basu (12 April 2020, London, United Kingdom)

'If physical gatherings – any kind of crowding – to protest become impossible, then the obvious way for protest to go would be into the digital space.'

Suman, I think that this statement privileges a certain space, social formation, and experience of registering protest over others. You might even be right in privileging physical gatherings – but I find it useful to ponder on this point to understand more about contemporary protests, anti-authoritarian actions, and collective action.

First, why are crowds as well as images and other representations of crowds important in a protest? The first thing that comes to mind is the issue of legitimacy in a public sphere. If we think this, then digital protests do much more than organizing this crowd – they transform the space of protest as well in a more substantial way. By representing this action on a platform with potentially global reach, as well as a discursive space with a different regulatory apparatus and regulation, it transforms the performative force of the act of crowding in a city square or a physical space.

I am careful to suggest here that it somehow exists outside the reach of state repressive apparatus, but it definitely brings in online witnesses to the equation who may or may not have been participants in first the instance of gathering in a crowd or witnessing a crowd or opposing a crowd. This could also, of course, extend to the actions of actors who react against the crowds or victims of state violence, as we saw in the video of Philando Castile in 2016[14] which sparked the Black Lives Matter movement.[15]

A lot more needs to be explored in the relationship between space and performativity in protest, including slogans. What happens to slogans when they move online? What happens to them when they are revived after decades? How are slogans different in different spaces, and what does that have to do with performativity? Is using a hashtag like #blacklivesmatter or #humdekhenge the same as chanting it in a crowd? Are slogan-hashtags different from other hashtags (like #newsnight)? The context-collapse that slogans face when taken online is definitely something to explore. And I think performativity is one way to explore it.

Second, picking up from your point 2 in this email, when it comes to online campaigning it is worth thinking again about what a successful or effective campaign is. And how do we measure this? As someone who has written numerous reports on campaigns as a marketing professional, I can tell you that the metrics really vary from campaign to campaign, although most clients' go-to is to look at simple platform-generated metrics like 'likes' or 'shares' or 'views', whatever it is on a particular platform. Agencies would often 'educate' clients to look beyond these metrics – and there are various tools that would allow you to do some crude sentiment and content analysis to measure the success of campaigns better. The main thing that clients want to see is a rise in whatever number, so agencies would pick whatever number rose most impressively and would try to show the growth over a period of time to justify a retainer. We have definitely seen a tendency to measure in a similar way the impact of research projects on communities in recent years. It is sufficient to say, then, that this trend is also being used to measure the success of digital campaigns in most of the recent literature on the topic.

As you have rightly pointed out in 2(ii), this is fairly meaningless – especially since we don't really know how many of these numbers actually matter in a given polity. 'Effective change', as we have seen in terms of the anti-Brexit petition and others, has been fairly few and far between. I am, however, sceptical about how far lectures, dharnas, and petitions can be said to have been directly effective over a shortish period of time. Instead I will suggest that these 'political tactics' have always been targeted at educating certain publics about issues of the day – like abolition, suffrage, imperialism, and so on. They have also been used as a way to show people's representatives in parliamentary democracies what certain publics want from them. I think that these function in a pretty similar way in their contemporary digitally mediated format – although who exactly signs these petitions, and who has access to this sort of political discourse, is, as you rightly point out, based on access. Where I don't agree with you is in your claim that the lack of immediate success of these petitions and their continued proliferation point towards them being tools of diffusing some frustration with the political system and the sense of powerlessness to effect any real change (although, of course, this does happen). What I want to say is that I don't think that the diffusion is the only thing happening or even the primary thing that is happening in these genres of political action.

I think that it is also an expression of desire to be part of the political decision-making, at least in issues that are important to one. It is also a way for one to fulfil one's desire to form some sort of collective around an issue that might not be seen as 'political'. The main point here is that the effectiveness of the campaign would be how far it allows these affective expectations of these publics to be satisfied and what happens when they are not satisfied. Here we see disappointment and defeat themselves act as perhaps a springboard of further politicization or creative interventions – definitely experience building in one's engagement with protest cultures. It allows one to come in contact with others in the same space, with life-changing or life-challenging experiences which shape one's worldview. It might at the very least allow them to form an idea of the issue as part of the collective and transcend their own experience of it. There is a strategic aspect to this but also a meaning-making and identity-related aspect. When does one start identifying as a black femme woman? And is this identity stable?

Notes

1 'Police entered Jamia Millia Islamia by force, students beaten up: Varsity', *India Today*, 15 December 2020, www.indiatoday.in/india/story/jamia-protest-against-cab-chief-proctor-statement-1628491-2019-12-15; Nehal Ahmed and Grace Raju, 'Two doctoral students at New Delhi's Jamia Millia Islamia recount December 15 police action to break their protest', *AlJazeera*, 18 December 2019, www.aljazeera.com/news/2019/12/heard-gunfire-jamia-students-detail-police-attack-campus-191218063347967.html; 'Jamia students and eyewitnesses recount the horrors of police violence' (video), *The Wire*, 16 December 2019, www.youtube.com/watch?v=FjKfY7_uWMs (accessed 30 May 2020).
2 Vijayta Lalwani, 'Why have Delhi and UP police blocked alternative routes around Shaheen Bagh?' *Scroll.in*, 10 February 2020, https://scroll.in/article/952617/why-have-delhi-and-up-police-blocked-alternative-routes-around-shaheen-bagh; 'Plea in Supreme Court over traffic blockade in Delhi's Shaheen Bagh', *Hindustan Times*, 20 January 2020, www.hindustantimes.com/cities/plea-in-sc-over-traffic-blockade-in-delhi-s-shaheen-bagh/story-t4y0HTc0LVdfT9rdcqWxBJ.html; Krishnadas Rajagopal, 'Shaheen Bagh closure: There cannot be indefinite protest in common area, says SC', *Hindu*, 10 February 2010, www.thehindu.com/news/national/shaheen-bagh-closure-there-cannot-be-indefinite-protest-in-common-area-says-sc/article30782154.ece?homepage=true; 'Shaheen Bagh mediator tells SC protest peaceful, police block roads', *India Today*, 23 February 2020, www.indiatoday.in/india/story/shaheen-bagh-interlocutor-sc-protest-peaceful-police-block-roads-1649193-2020-02-23 (accessed 30 May 2020).
3 Arvind Ojha, 'Shaheen Bagh firing: Shooter shouts sirf Hinduon ki chalegi, detained', *India Today*, 1 February 2020, www.indiatoday.in/india/story/shaheen-bagh-shooting-anti-caa-protest-violence-delhi-police-protesters-1642353-2020-02-01; Munish Chandra Pandey, 'Jamia shooter self-radicalised, took part in Bajrang Dal rally, reveals initial probe', *India Today*, 31 January 2020, www.indiatoday.in/india/story/jamia-shooter-self-radicalised-took-part-in-bajrang-dal-rally-1641855-2020-01-31 (accessed 30 May 2020).
4 Gustave Le Bon, *The Crowd: A Study of the Popular Mind* (Kitchener: Batoshe Books, 2001 [1869]); Elias Canetti, *Crowds and Power* (Harmondsworth: Penguin, 1960); Philip Zimbardo, 'The human choice: Individuation, reason and order versus deindividuation, impulse and chaos', in W.J. Arnold and D. Levine, eds. *Nebraska Symposium on Motivation* (Lincoln: University of Nebraska Press, 1969).

5 Mark Easton, 'Coronavirus: Significant minority find lockdown "extremely difficult", poll suggests', *BBC*, 9 April 2020, www.bbc.com/news/uk-52228169 (accessed 30 May 2020).

6 Faisal Islam, 'Record fall in UK economy forecast', *BBC*, 9 April 2020, www.bbc.com/news/business-52232639 (accessed 30 May 2020).

7 See Chapter 2, endnote 7.

8 'Brazil's health ministry has 76% approval rating; Bolsonaro, 33%', *Folha de S.Paulo*, 6 April 2020, https://www1.folha.uol.com.br/internacional/en/brazil/2020/04/brazils-health-ministry-has-76-approval-rating-bolsonaro-33.shtml (accessed 30 May 2020). Bolsonaro's approval rating went up despite higher ratings for Health Minister Mandetta after he gave a seemingly conciliatory television address on 31 March: ' "We're facing the biggest challenge of our generation", Bolsonaro says', *Agência Brasil*, 1 April 2020, https://agenciabrasil.ebc.com.br/en/politica/noticia/2020-04/were-facing-biggest-challenge-our-generation-bolsonaro-says; Daniel Carvalho and Fábio Fabrini, 'Bolsonaro says Brazil's mission is to save lives without losing jobs in televised public address', *Folha de S.Paulo*, 1 April 2020, https://www1.folha.uol.com.br/internacional/en/brazil/2020/04/bolsonaro-says-brazils-mission-is-to-save-lives-without-losing-jobs-in-televised-public-address.shtml (accessed 1 June 2020).

9 'Tentativa de cassar registro do PT é perseguição política', 9 April 2020, www.youtube.com/watch?v=DCRjiq2yYEs (accessed 1 June 1990).

10 'Милен Велчев: 10-те млрд. дълг не са предназначени за незабавно харчене', programme 'Денят започва с Георги Любенов', *BNT 1*, 11 April 2020, www.bnt.bg/bg/a/milen-velchev-10-te-mlrd-dlg-ne-sa-prednaznacheni-za-nezabavno-kharchene#recap (accessed 30 May 2020).

11 'Petition: Revoke Article 50 and remain in the EU', got 6,103,056 signatures and was debated on 1 April 2019, https://petition.parliament.uk/archived/petitions/241584 (accessed 30 May 2020).

12 Let me note as an aside that 'non-profit' and 'social enterprise' are both vague terms and may not be quite as conscience driven and indifferent to finance as many may think.

13 See https://petition.parliament.uk/ (accessed 30 May 2020).

14 'Philando Castile police shooting video livestreamed on Facebook', *ABC News*, 7 July 2016, www.youtube.com/watch?v=PEjipYKbOOU (accessed 30 May 2020).

15 See https://blacklivesmatter.com/ (accessed 30 May 2020).

6

THE POOR AND THE WAY OUT

Summary: *As the initial deadlines for lockdowns drew near, in various countries patience with inactivity and enclosure was wearing thin. There was little to justify any quick relaxation of restrictions, but the economic pressures mounted and with them the demands for relaxation. The effect of the lockdowns on those in precarious or straitened circumstances was much in the news and on the authors' minds. The interventions in this chapter touch upon those tensions. These tensions were, naturally, both external and internal — in various ways, the interventions here are as much on tensions observed out there as on the authors' own unsettled feelings.*

Suman Gupta (12 April 2020, Delhi, India)

Milena's fantasy switching-off protest reminds me of José Saramago's novel *Seeing*, which has an electorate which simply refuses to vote decisively one way or another in the general elections, with a majority casting blank votes, leading gradually to the declaration of a state of emergency and the imposition of authoritarian rule and lockdown. And that reminds me that *Seeing* is a sequel to *Blindness*, which is in fact about a mysterious epidemic which makes the population of a city blind and leads to social collapse.

But let's pause on the present.

Yesterday an altercation among the Delhi homeless in locked-down shelters led to three shelters being burnt down.[1] An older group in the shelters felt that the quality of the food they were receiving (from donors, apparently) had dropped after a new set of arrivals.

We are at an interesting juncture, aren't we? All those leaders are talking about 'relaxation' and 'exit strategy' even in the United States, United Kingdom, Spain, and Italy, with very thin or no rays of hope in those two big figures: the accruing tally of confirmed cases and of deaths (okay, we have stopped worrying about recoveries). The same talk here in India, too. There are extensions of lockdown but tired, nervous extensions. WHO is saying that loosening lockdowns could lead to a devastating resurgence of infections.[2]

This is a bit like checking the tensile strength of a material by stretching and bending it. The lockdown is a gradually increasing weight, checking how far it can go. The idea is to go as far as possible *without* breaking the stuff being stretched — how to describe that? 'Social fabric' according to sociologists and social scientists; 'the economy' according to political and business gurus. How far can one go without breaking this stuff? This is an impossible question. A materials scientist knows what the tensile strength of a material is by taking it to the breaking point, by letting it break and measuring that point. If this material being tested by the lockdown has to stop short of breaking and we don't know when it could break, how short or long should one stop?

Nevertheless, the lockdown stretching has put longstanding things into perspective — thrown them into sharp relief — where they have otherwise tended to pass amidst habituated indifference. One of the things that can obviously stretch too far and shouldn't, to the breaking point, is unemployment and poverty. Fear of poverty is a constant motive force for politics and economics, though no one really measures the breaking point thereof — they focus on the upbeat factors that describe the affluent worldview while extirpating that driving fear. Fear of poverty has become the explicit theme of lockdown economics. How many are going to be unemployed, how many will lose their homes, how many will sink into depression, how many small businesses will become bankrupt, how many benefit-seekers to be added, how big the recession. . . . The lockdown economy tries to stave off that fear for as long as possible, by promises of short-term compensation, providing shelter and food, considering bailouts for a while but after having fallen out of the means and systems for doing so regularly and as a matter of course. So, all this sounds panicky, merely an anticipation of and desperation about more poverty. Fifty million may be added to those in poverty in India, it was reported the day before. Images of migrant labourers walking without food or water trying to get out of locked-down cities, where there's no living any longer, for the impoverished homes they left; street vendors being beaten into lockdown, their wares being upturned by policemen (the sort of thing that marked the beginning of dramatic protests in Tunisia in December 2010)[3] — these images on Indian TV have stirred a new kind of fear — a heightened fear of poverty and the poor. This is evinced in exaggerated and shrill charitable pronouncements and recriminations, forgetting that in fact these images are merely an accentuation of an everyday reality; street vendors are treated more or less in that way every day somewhere, migrant labourers have the most precarious lives on the edge. . . . In the United States and therefore by rote in the United Kingdom, as the night the day, it is found that the ethnic minorities (which mainly means 'black' and 'brown', who are mainly poorer) are the most vulnerable and need to be especially vigilant — it's in the news. But it has ever been so, only now it seems like news. In the United States earlier this month, it was reported that over 6 million have registered unemployed,[4] but that number will soon be doubled or quadrupled. In India, the appearance of the contagion in the largest slum in Asia, Dharavi in Mumbai, alongside two or three other slum areas, sounds like a particularly ominous death knell.[5] Meanwhile, no one in India is more culpable now than the Muslim organization Tablighi Jamaat for spreading the virus in India[6] – it was all within control so long as rich cosmopolitan people were spreading the virus from their foreign visits and high-profile contacts. And yet this is how, in general, things have been for a while: the poor get the worst deal from any government act (demonetization in 2016 a good recent example), and Muslims are always more culpable than anyone else in India in this brave new millennium.

So, fear of poverty – that's a push for talk about 'an exit strategy' and 'relaxation' before any specific condition for the lockdown itself has been clearly alleviated yet. That fear could be an anticipation of this sort of argument: the risk of dying from coronavirus is put at under 5% by most experts; the risk of living a life-not-worth-living in poverty and deprivation and dying that way seems now around 80% – what's there to lose by starting an anti-social-distancing crowd protest? We don't want to get to the critical proportion of any population coming up with that argument.

But there's another side to this juncture, too, this premature or all-too-necessary – depending how you see it – talk about an 'exit strategy' and 'relaxation' before anything decisive about the contagion can be demonstrated. It's a portent of making uncertainty and the contagion perpetual. There's a contagion that's always there at large to some degree, and we are nevertheless working in its midst. We need to be ever vigilant forever; some degree of emergency condition has to be maintained perpetually so that relaxation from emergency is also perpetual.

Milena Katsarska (12 April 2020, Plovdiv, Bulgaria)

Although Bulgaria is indeed a petri dish in comparison to India and other countries, both the juncture described and the apprehensions and talk are exactly the same. I guess, from the perspective of a locked-down country, these are inevitably what come up: the threat of poverty from within and vulnerable and minority groups as the threatening other.

This was clear in yesterday's messages here, whereby the 'operational headquarters' (the medical military team of experts) made it clear that there's no practical logic that would justify an easing or relaxation of the regime, that is, in terms of reasoning from what is known of the spread of Covid-19.[7] That position is directly contradicted now by the government and political/economic elites for the reasons you outline. In countries where they wheeled out a crisis management team that is not aligned with or composed of the rulers of the day, that will create a juncture at which attempts will be made to renegotiate the position of that crisis management team or to dismiss it. For now, Boyko is too scared to do that, I think. Actually, in my view, he is panicking because everything is way beyond him personally, while he's been trying to hold the fort and fill all holes precisely as a personality. In fact, now that I think about it, there's a third option at the top of current governing arrangements, and that is in the General (now one of the three leaders in Bulgaria) who is a surgeon and a military man. I suppose he could get angry and resign from the top position of the crisis headquarters managing team. Incidentally, the other two leaders are also generals – Prime Minister Borisov himself (an interior ministry general) and President Radev (a pilot military general). Should there be any doubt – Bulgaria is indeed led by generals.[8]

Moves in the direction of relaxation with conditions are already evident. The first 'easy' condition verbalized is that 'the elderly' will stay in isolation for a year. This caught my eye somewhere in print. That ticks several boxes; that's why it is the easy option. (1) This is a demographic which, by and large, at least on paper, has a small but steady regular income based on retirement plans, with allegedly no active productive role in the economy. However, none of this is quite so clear cut. (2) This is also the demographic which all can feel a moral responsibility for keeping safe and feeling charitable towards, as a good civil society. I wonder what other arguments can be put forward to carve out other groups based on a similar logic that would be just as agreeable so as to start painting the picture of the new normal. Generally, it is quite easy to remove the so-called social groups that are already on the edge of visibility.

One can foresee possible new modes of socializing by considering the reformatting of education that is taking place. We might be moving towards a generation that actually goes through a process of almost total 'online socialization' for educational purposes, starting with pragmatic compulsion and settling into habit and the-way-things-are. Arguably, the only physical and social proximity that this generation would feel they need might turn out to be an occasional parental or sibling hug, strictly within the confines of kinship and domicile.

John Seed (12 April 2020, London, United Kingdom)

It's a beautiful spring weekend here – warm sunshine, blue skies, birds singing, blossoms thick on the trees.

The original strategy of 'herd immunity' (a term redolent of eugenics?) was always the only viable one in the long term. Lockdown was an emergency measure which will only delay the inevitable but will at least slow the process down. I suppose this can give medical facilities some possibility of coping. I heard a doctor in London the other day say that the situation in his hospital was like a major disaster incident but one that's happening every day. Two additional advantages of lockdown and thus slowing (delaying) the incidence of cases: treatment should become more effective as different strategies and drugs are trialled, and a vaccine may become available. However, I don't think vaccines can provide a long-term magic cure. Apparently, the virus is mutating quite rapidly, as viruses generally do. So any vaccine will have limited effectiveness, as flu vaccines always do. A vaccine will help, obviously, but within shifting limits. On the same principle, incidentally, immunity from having had the virus will be only partial in the longer term.

The virus is here to stay for the foreseeable future and for the vast majority of the population is just another unpleasant flu virus. For the older and those with pre-existing health conditions, it's now an additional hazard and will shorten life expectancy for years to come. I expect the next 12–18 months will be a fluctuating scenario: relaxation of social distancing, reopening of schools and shops, spikes in cases and deaths, a short-term return of restrictions, further relaxations, and so on. So we can indeed expect a new normal: face masks will become common on city streets, fear of the other will be intensified, and sociability will be overshadowed by a phobia around touching. I expect the older will withdraw even further from social life into a mild paranoia. Going to the theatre or a town centre or any social gathering will have additional risks. Risk society or wot!

As for the sociology of Covid-19: yes, obviously the poorer you are, the more vulnerable you will be to infection because of conditions of everyday life – living in crowded conditions where social distancing and scrupulous hygiene are impossible, pushing up against each other in stuffy crowded buses, eating a poorer diet, engaging in long hours of exhausting and unhealthy work. Covid-19 simply reveals pre-existing health inequalities. I saw some US figures on the significantly higher black death rate.[9] Some preliminary statistics seem to indicate that in the United Kingdom, there is a higher incidence of being badly affected by the virus among black Caribbean and Asian groups.[10] However, you shouldn't reach for a simple correlation between ethnicities and poverty and therefore greater vulnerability to Covid-19. There are other determinants in play here.

Thus, for instance, higher incidence of diabetes among those groups, for instance, is not a simple effect of poverty. Cheap mass-produced food full of carbohydrates is one major factor in causing diabetes and metabolic syndrome (pre-diabetes/obesity). I suspect these medical conditions are higher among Asian and Caribbean groups. But fresh fruit and vegetables are just as cheap. And the white working class are as prone to diabetes and pre-diabetes and obesity. A London perspective can easily miss this. Were the sex ratios of deaths – 73% male and 27% female[11] – reversed, we might have been concerned about gender inequality. Maybe men are more likely to smoke and indulge in other unhealthy pleasures. They are certainly much more likely to engage in unhealthy work. Or maybe there's a biological factor increasing male mortality. I saw some research that suggested that some blood groups (not 'O') were more vulnerable. So ethnicity and class and biology and material environment and diet and lifestyle choices, and so on are interconnected in complicated ways. The life expectancy of a working-class man in Glasgow not long ago was under 50. If this was an effect of poverty, it was realized in very specific ways.

The brick wall that socialist governments of every kind have banged their head against generation after generation is now on the agenda like never before. The poorest people often seem to have a death wish and despite every measure and attempt at education will engage in behaviour which will make their life worse.

Now, if you wish not to suffer badly from this virus – and even die – you need to stop smoking, lose weight, stop booze and drugs, and change your diet. It's not only about the direct effects of material poverty but also about their leisure activities! Yes, I know, it's the old spectre of the lumpenproletariat and I sound like every old labour activist and old Bolshevik. And yes, this kind of argument can be used – and probably will be used – to justify different social and ethnic (and gender?) outcomes of Covid-19 in terms of mortality. But the medical experts will have a point when they provide hard and indisputable evidence that if you smoke, are diabetic or pre-diabetic and obese – consequences of a bad diet and lifestyle – you are more likely to die of Covid-19, just as you are more likely to die pre-Covid-19 of other illnesses. Let's hope this issue does not disguise the bigger issues of bad housing, low wages, and unhealthy work and material environment which also make a huge contribution to differential mortality of classes. I suppose 1945 was one precedent of how a more or less socialist party managed the transition from a war economy to peace, using devastation to create a better economy and state for the majority of the population. Any such possibility of a good outcome in Britain in 2020–21 seems remote.

The discontent with the effects of lockdown that you begin to detect might well develop into a tidal wave of riot and disorder in some parts of the world. But what kind of political project will inform it? That's a bigger question. The old Bolshevik in me thinks that without the leadership of a radical and intelligent political party, that anger will merely target vulnerable scapegoats and symbols and will destroy but not change anything very much. The US Democrats also seem to have a death wish, so we can expect four more years of Trump unless he drops dead. We have four more years of the Tories here, and looking across the channel at Europe, there's a political wasteland. The EU is going to suffer some bitter divisions around Covid-19. To nobody's surprise, Germany immediately closed its borders and seems to have left the Italians and Spanish to deal with things on their own.[12] The Chinese offered more practical help than Berlin or Brussels.[13] More fodder for the nationalist right to feed on. Anyway, the fallout of Covid-19 is going to shape EU politics too for the next few years.

Peter H. Tu (12 April 2020, Niskayuna, New York State, United States)

These are odd times. Trump has a talent for saying what other politicians are surely thinking but dare not utter: 'The cure might be worse that the disease'.[14] The threat of 1930s-style poverty brought on by a worldwide depression seems most unpalatable. But one can't help but feel that the poor are not the ones tugging at Trump's heartstrings; rather, it is the oligarchs who need the masses to be harnessed and tethered to the machines of production in order to keep their fortunes afloat.

For re-election purposes, Trump was planning to thump his chest over a triumphant economy. Oddly enough, consolidation of power with the goal of authoritarianism does not seem to be taking place in the US. Instead, Trump is doing as much as he can not to take responsibility for anything. He says that the states and not the federal government must be the ones to find the resources needed to fight this virus. He fears putting down any form of national shelter-in-place directive, probably because his state news agency Fox has made rural voters feel that this is an urban problem. . . . The hardest-hit states like New York and New Jersey are told that they must make do with the ventilators and PPE that they have, while swing states such as Florida and Kentucky are denied nothing.[15] One of the great villains of the Trump regime is his trade advisor Peter Navarro – he seems to be behind much of the politicization of the Covid-19 crisis.[16] You might have seen the spectacle in Wisconsin.[17] The Democrat governor wanted to postpone the primary elections; the Republican state senators would have none of it. The governor then tried for a mail-in ballot, and the Republicans howled against this as well – they fear anything that makes it easier to vote. The US Supreme Court, now firmly in Republican hands, sided solidly with their Republican brothers. So Wisconsiners had to line up for hours to vote. Most of the poll operators are elderly volunteers, so many of them did not show up. As a consequence, Milwaukee, one of the largest cities in Wisconsin, only had four operational polling stations. . . . Well I could go on and on about this type of craziness.

So how do we get things going again? In some ways, Covid-19 feels a bit like the old Roman practice of decimation. One in 10 of those that are infected will end up being hospitalized, and maybe 1 in 5 will not survive. It is kind of like being given a bag of Skittles with the mild warning that one or two of those candies are poisonous – most of us would forego the pleasure of such treats. And so we shelter in place. Part of me also wonders if this is an opportunity to rethink things in general. It seems to me that certain life-sustaining industries are more Covid-19 resistant than others. Agriculture and rural life (at least in the West) are pretty much a mechanized and somewhat solitary affair, and so are our distribution systems. In fact, at this time, farms are having to destroy produce because demand is so low. The same might be said for energy production and construction. Factories, offices, and warehouses seem to sit in the middle. They could be turned into low-risk sites via a combination of: screening, cleaning, PPE, social-distance policy, and teleworking when possible. What seems problematic are: schools, childcare, mass transit (I have been in many meetings trying to figure out what it would take to get people to feel safe enough to fly again), travel in general, tourism, restaurants, hotels. . . . Maybe we have a new reason for the rise of robots. I guess in general the tech solutions will be: efficient methods for testing, the ability to track down those that have come in contact with the infected, treatments for those that have been infected, and, of course, a vaccine. On the bright side, it can be argued that the number of lives saved due to reductions in pollution, car accidents, and influenza is larger than the number of Covid-19 deaths.

I guess in this context, we have to consider parallels and intersections with climate change. This problem, where we are aware of the risks but refuse to prepare until it is too late, seems to be a fundamental crisis of international leadership. There is a bit of a tragedy of the commons thing going on here – everyone needs to cooperate in order to make this thing go away. If in January, when the always very bad Chinese finally admitted that things had gone awry, the whole world had done the unthinkable – just shelter in place for two weeks – we would have been rid of this thing once and for all. The worldwide shelter-in-place that we are now under feels a bit like a drowning world getting a short gasp of air. The sad thing is that the four trillion dollars that the US is printing to keep things going could have in theory paid for the electrification of the entire country. And, of course, Bernie Sanders has exited stage left[18] – we now have to pin our hopes on an age-ing Joe Biden, who is in the process of empathizing with everyone from his lonely basement.

As for living like this, there seem to be some hard choices ahead. My brother is a general practitioner and supports many of Vancouver's homeless population. He is basically resigned to the idea that Covid-19 will simply have its way with this community – it will be like a wildfire, take its toll, and then be over. I hear this sentiment from countries in Africa where droughts, war, and other calamities make Covid-19 look like a walk in the park by comparison. I suppose the refugee camps and slums in general are similarly doomed.

As for myself, in early January, in anticipation of what was to come, we bought a large freezer. I made sure that the money I saved to pay for the children's university (a significant cost in the United States) was pulled out of the stock markets. Since my funding comes from the government, for the next 15 months my employment is relatively secure. As far as I can tell, the very definition of the suburbs is social distancing. Both A and J are taking their lessons via the Internet, which also serves as our source of entertainment and interaction with the outside world. But at the end of the day, this is a prison, and I want out.

Milena Katsarska (12 April 2020, Plovdiv, Bulgaria)

Exchanged greetings on the phone with people who have their Name Day today. Mainly heard depressed people: there's some sense of a grave tightening of the situation, whereby masks have become obligatory as of midnight.

This evening I decided to listen to the online morning briefing that I had missed. Well, this was really something. If there was any doubt about the emergency head-quarters' abdication or dismissal, that was put to rest. The ranks of medical profes-sionals have presented a united front that could scare zombies back to oblivion. Apparently, there was some laid-back behaviour by people in the capital yesterday, with people just going into 'fuck-it' mode and walking about boulevards, parks, and so on in joyful abandon under the sun, getting ready for the religious holiday today. So, this morning, our main protagonist the General wheeled out the head of the Medical Association, three major Sofia hospital directors, and so on. They produced an unprecedented sermon for the unsuspecting (or suspecting) citizens of this country. I don't think I've ever heard a top doctor addressing the nation live on national TV about God, and how He is with each and every one at home on an everyday basis – so, don't go to church or anywhere for the designated holiday! He then proceeded to detail what his surgery routine for 27 years has been every time he went into an operation, because doctors need to believe too, and that has been shaped as a fatalistic ritual of sorts. Then the rest of the medical representatives present declared their status of being delegated by the medical community of the country (nurses and doctors) who had written to urge them to speak on their behalf with the message: 'Keep us – medical professionals – safe with responsible behaviour, so that we can continue to do our jobs, which is a no mean deal', and 'if you do so, we will be the ones clapping at 8 pm'. The on-air accounts of these gents (all men) did not spare a single gory detail of the videos exchanged within medical networks; with everyday matter-of-factness they talked of counts and the availability of body bags, of a mother who was denied the right to bury her son (one of several such cases here), of counting freezer capacity and checking whether and how fast a canteen freezer can be refurbished to the aim of body storage. . . . Now that explains the depressed colleagues I had spoken to earlier. But I also admired this briefing: there's the unvarnished brutal truth, not some rhetorical ploy by some politician or other.

Boyko's relaxation ideas were effectively axed at the ankles with this. In a perverse way, I'm quite enjoying this daily drama. The main protagonist of our story, the General, has proven his intelligence yet again. Following the narrative, I had him pegged as an atheist. So he invited others, with whom he shares a professional domain, to the table, and they delivered a most striking united front to scare Bulgarians – probably because Bulgarians need doses of fear; I don't know.

Onwards . . . today was both Palm Sunday (Orthodox style) and Easter Sunday (Catholic style). It didn't really matter that 'the temples' were open. I have not heard a whiff of anything being celebrated within 100 yards of a church. And then I heard about the closure of the farmers' markets for the day. Those markets will be allowed to work Monday through Wednesday and will be closed indefinitely thereafter. Then the prime minister (also being a general) has ordered the social services to use government money to buy all the locally produced veggies and fruits that would be left to rot otherwise because of the closure and to distribute them among vulnerable people for the holidays. How exactly that will happen, we don't really know, but it will be done because Boyko has said so.

Richard Allen (13 April 2020, Birmingham, United Kingdom)

It seems more than redundant to say that Easter here isn't quite normal. We're not churchgoers, but it's part of the Englishness of where we live that there is a church just round the corner, so we hear the bells regularly. It's all quiet this year. It's also a little unusual in that it is rather warm and sunny. It's not at all unusual for there to be a bit of snow around at Easter, especially when it falls early. I well remember my friend from Kerala coming to stay and arriving at this time. We took him out into the countryside where there were patches of snow, which led to what one could only call frolicking in the strangeness on his part. G and I are both well and have settled into a kind of routine which involves usually a morning walk around our local – closed – golf course and the streets to get our paper before returning to our isolation. We have also become 'zoomers' for socializing and for G's yoga. I get out to my allotment – it's a busy time there. In truth, however, it is a bit boring. Lots of cultural organizations are organizing online events, to the extent that one can't keep up, which leaves one feeling a bit feeble!

There's also a sense of being a spectator at a very very slow car crash as one watches the failure of the government to manage things. There is excessive use of the future tense – 'there will be enough testing/equipment' – and of the aspirational – 'we are committed absolutely'. The *Guardian* tries in its moderate way to puncture this a bit now,[19] but otherwise the major feat of the government has been to conceal the fact that they were the government when all the lack of preparation went on. It's perhaps not on the Trump scale, but certainly other countries seem to be faring better – without always exercising a dictatorial fiat. The BBC regularly reports nurses saying they lack equipment/drugs, and so on.[20] And the government saying that there is now enough of the same without attempting to use its journalists to find out the facts/truth.

And there is talk of easing the lockdown to save the economy by those who show their real interests. There must come a time when the lockdown is eased, and that will be before there is a vaccine so that we will continue along the plateau in the number of deaths, but there's no sign at the moment that there are any who are ready to lead a moral discussion as opposed to expressing their self-interest. The situation is also revealing a startling inability amongst statisticians to do more than come up with headlines of a dubious kind, aided and abetted again by the BBC, and so on. The standard line goes: (1) 'the daily figure for the number of deaths is not reliable in terms of determining a trend or even telling you how many people actually died that day'; (2) with scarcely a pause for breath, let's speculate on the basis of this statistic which I have just undermined!

I can't, sitting in the calm of our detached house with a garden and with green spaces around us, think what it must be like for people stuck in flats, let alone people in poverty stuck in sub-standard flats or people stuck in sub-standard flats with an abusive partner . . . or what it's like in the population density of various parts of Delhi. Presumably, it is warming up now, so I hope electricity is available for coolers, and so on. I always remember when I stayed in Mumbai for a while and was able to use a flat on the 23rd floor of one of the tower blocks in Colaba. Looking out, one saw, more readily than when one arrived, the slums circling the base of the blocks – not to mention Dharavi. One can imagine the Indian government eradicating a disease in places like that, as they did with polio, but not managing any of the now-conventional wisdom about coronavirus – social distancing, infection tracing, and so on!

Fabio Akcelrud Durão (13 April 2020, São Carlos, São Paulo State, Brazil)

Suman, your musings on the physics of poverty and the resilience of the social tissue touch on what is for me the most important question now. I would only add to the equation the question of distribution of wealth. To what extent can the idea of redistribution of wealth be kept at bay? How easy is it not to mention that the superrich should provide the lion's share of the funding for economic readjustment?

The situation in Brazil is now different from India. As a result of economic necessity, exhaustion from confinement, and Bolsonaro's public statements, the quarantine is being prematurely softened. It is now estimated that countrywide less than 50% of the people are safely locked in their homes. So, we can brace ourselves here for a steep worsening of the contagion and number of cases. The Bolsonaro lot have now concentrated their attacks on the TV network Rede Globo – irony of ironies; this has been one of the most pernicious institutions in Brazil, together with the police and the military.[21] For my whole adult life, I dreamed of the Globo headquarters blowing up some day, since those days when I passed in front of them every day on the bus to school in Rio. Now Globo, without ceasing to be a baleful agent of domination, is the target of Bolsonaro, because he favours Record, owned by the fundamentalist church Universal, which is Brazil's biggest multinational corporation.[22]

All of this is to say that I suspect that Bolsonaro's tactic is to let people die in public hospitals (private ones are so far coping well with the epidemic) and not let it become socially visible. I don't know if this is feasible, but it may be the plan, if there is one. The situation is so bizarre that you can imagine a character in a novel saying: 'After all, 1% of the population is not so great a number, especially if mainly the elderly and weak are going to die. Two million individuals less is not something that would cripple the economy, on the contrary, it could invigorate it, like a medieval blood-letting, creating jobs and alleviating social security'. The question is to know how the families will react to these deaths. At any rate, we have to wait for the numbers, both of casualties and financial collapse, to consolidate.

Suman Gupta (13 April 2020, Delhi, India)

Though the first phase of the national lockdown is due to end tomorrow, there has been no announcement yet whether it will be extended. It would be considerate for these things to be announced sooner rather than later so that all can prepare themselves, at least mentally. This lockdown was announced four hours before it started; maybe they are trying to do it two hours before this time. If there's a reason behind this indecision, it could be to do partly with the federal structure of government and partly with contrary pulls of reluctance and necessity. A nationwide lockdown should be declared by the central government (Modi will appear on TV looking holier than anyone ever), a regional state lockdown by the relevant state government (the chief minister will appear on TV looking holier than thou but not as holy as Modi). Some state governments – Odisha, West Bengal, Punjab – have already declared extensions of the lockdown to the end of the month. I think so has Maharashtra, where Mumbai is the eye of the storm. Delhi will, too, because it's the other eye of the storm, but no one has said so yet. The question is: would there be an extension of the national lockdown?

Or is keeping some states locked down and letting others choose for themselves the first phase of relaxation?

The policy in Delhi and Mumbai, meanwhile, is to establish containment zones around spots where infected persons have been found – a kind of cordon sanitaire. Areas of within a kilometre square are sealed in. In this area, no one is allowed to step out of their homes unless there's a medical emergency (if you step out, it had better be bad enough so that it might be stepping out for good). Essential food is delivered by government-appointed personnel. Such containment is kept in place until it is clear that there are no more infections in that area. I'm not sure how that's worked out – whether they just wait for more cases, and if there're none within 14 days, they remove the barriers, or whether they get down to testing everyone. Reports suggest that such containment has been characteristically ham-handed and inefficient in the first instance – police at the gates of sealed areas have turned away doctors who had turned up to do screening, food has not been delivered, and so on.[23]

Testing everyone is a fraught matter, but only partly because there aren't test kits or adequate equipment and protection for health workers. That's also because people are often hostile to health workers and doctors. In various places, starting from Indore and then in various cities around the country, mobs have attacked health workers sent to screen local populations, pelting them with stones.[24] In hospitals, doctors and nurses have been abused, beaten, and spat at.[25] A couple of women doctors out buying vegetables in Delhi were manhandled.[26] Landlords are asking health workers who are tenants to vacate their premises or are refusing to let homes to them.[27] The Delhi government issued a notice at the end of March saying that such landlords will be prosecuted.[28] In some parts of town, reportedly, drones are being deployed to check where people with high temperatures are in congested areas, possibly to spray disinfectants on these concentrated masses.

My part of town hasn't been sealed in yet, so I can go shopping and for a brisk walk in the evening. The temperatures are now creeping towards 40 degrees C, promised today, and face masks (or some sort of covering) have been compulsory for a week or so – a face mask in a Delhi summer is no joke. Not many people go for a walk. One mainly meets street vegetable vendors looking stoical, ragged street children, and some middle-class persons in their masks with shopping bags hurrying along purposefully. But that's on the main street. In the *basti* not far off, and in the long narrow lanes of formerly unauthorized colonies (about the width of two of me standing side by side), there are people who can't get away from each other and therefore don't really try. I can see gatherings in the distance there, and I think I even saw a bazaar in progress up one alley but pretended not to see it and hurried along. Typically Delhi police are few, far between, indifferent or scowling, in this part of town. The middle-class cooperative blocks have locked themselves in like fortresses and have banned all day-working servants (all middle-class households have servants to clean floors, wash dishes, do any heavy lifting, and be general dogsbody). I suppose the middle-class people – especially women – are keeping themselves occupied some of the day doing *all* the housework, which must be a novel experience. I hope they are carrying on paying their absent army of informal domestic labour until they can get back to work; otherwise they are all in serious trouble. This army is employed on word-of-mouth agreements, their work as quickly disposable as it is flexible.

Milena Katsarska (13 April 2020, Plovdiv, Bulgaria)

I am beginning to see deep differences within my circle of friends. R is treading an unreasonable furrow now, in my view, half-buying into conspiracy theories and lapsing into righteous anger at the government's evident attempts to be logical. Last night he went on a texting ramble about the 'apathy of the general population' regarding the closure of farmers' markets. The thing is that nobody in the higher echelons actually thinks that closing said markets is an unproblematic idea, but it is perhaps a move that is necessary, as those had become contagion hotspots. The problem is that the moment one announces such a measure, one has to have in place (already) an action plan for the farmers and their existing produce. This is not about emotions but about lack of foresight and planning – such moves cannot be announced out of the blue, without an a, b, c to fall back on. The temporary 'solution' was to have them open until Wednesday to ensure the movement of said produce, but that of course doesn't solve the problem of further local produce ripening and getting ready to be sold. There's a degree of nationalism in this as well, and protectionism, because it is local producers who are foregrounded as the main concern, not importers or retailers of local veggies and fruit, who are also losing out. For this conundrum to be solved without nationalism muddying the waters, or righteous indignation about 'our very own' hard-working agrarians, three days are not nearly enough. That should have been considered well in advance.

Then, of course, that scenario has a clear Sofia-feel to it, and I can see now how the Sofia vs countryside divide is about to blow up big time. It was in Sofia that both the markets disregarded the measures blatantly, just as it was Sofia residents who defiantly milled and clustered as the weekend approached. If anything, I see a liberal middle-class unruliness and lower-middle-class nationalist defiance in the making. Lumpen politicians (for lack of a better word) and other fringe or not-so-fringe populists of different hues are coming up with calls 'for protests', while there are also hefty online generators of conspiracy theories. R is half-buying into the latter. In a phone conversation with M last night, I realized that she is worried big time because her son is lapping those up wholesale. She got wind of a network organization for travelling to Sofia to 'make some noise' in the streets and 'take down the government'.

This is just the tip of the iceberg of stupidity, in my view. This has dimensions of individual unthinkingness and mass gullibility in probably equal measure. All this unfolded while I was just beginning to detect what I thought were optimistic local signs in the direction of let's call it 'prospective socialism'. Something like that is, in fact, achievable here given the miniscule scale of Bulgaria, its relative containment, not insurmountable class gaps, and so on. The preconditions are in fact all there, and amusingly enough, the current leadership (in the person of spokesman Boyko) is apparently inclined to resort to such kind of thinking in the face of a crisis. He had indeed announced a per-person aid package for people who were on 20-day non-paid leaves for April to the amount for 345 or 375 leva the other day, contrary to our neoliberal financiers' advice.[29] That was among other moves to expand 'social packages' to encompass larger portions of the population. It is probably due to this glimmer of budging towards direct state care at the ground level (not just big businesses or business per se) that those old spectres of red terror were deliberately stirred again, and the neoliberal elites, like the nationalist populists, are ready to pounce.

It is probably fair to say that any crisis brings forth and throws into relief precisely those contextual nuances that are already there. That's not just on the surface, in terms of what was going on immediately before the crisis struck, but also in a deep structure of ideas, inclinations, and firmly entrenched dispositions with a long historical shadow.

Notes

1 'Three shelters housing 150 gutted, Delhi cops point at food row', *Times of India*, 12 April 2020, https://timesofindia.indiatimes.com/city/delhi/3-shelters-housing-150-people-gutted-cops-point-at-food-row/articleshow/75102461.cms (accessed 30 May 2020).

2 Sarah Wheaton, 'WHO chief: Lifting lockdowns early risks "deadly resurgence"', *Politico*, 10 April 2020, www.politico.eu/article/who-chief-speedy-lockdown-lifts-risk-deadly-resurgence/ (accessed 30 May 2020).

3 For an account, see: Suman Gupta, Milena Katsarska, Theodoros Spyros, and Mike Hajimichael, *Usurping Suicide: The Political Resonances of Individual Deaths* (London: Zed, 2017), Ch.2.

4 Dominic Rushe and Lauren Aratani, 'Coronavirus batters US economy as 6.65m file for unemployment last week', *Guardian*, 2 April 2020, www.theguardian.com/business/2020/apr/02/us-unemployment-coronavirus-economy (accessed 30 May 2020).

5 Tanvi Deshpande, 'Coronavirus – Dharavi emerges as COVID-19 hotspot', *Hindu*, 2 April 2020, www.thehindu.com/news/cities/mumbai/coronavirus-bmc-sweeper-is-second-positive-case-in-dharavi/article31234805.ece (accessed 30 May 2020).

6 Saurabh Trivedi, 'Coronavirus – The story of India's largest COVID-19 cluster', *Hindu,* 11 April 2020, www.thehindu.com/news/national/coronavirus-nizamuddin-tablighi-jamaat-markaz-the-story-of-indias-largest-covid-19-cluster/article31313698.ece; Rizwan Ahmad, 'Media watch: How vocabulary was weaponised to target Indian Muslims after the Tablighi Jamat event', *Scroll.in*, 12 April 2020, https://scroll.in/article/958976/media-watch-how-vocabulary-was-weaponised-to-target-indian-muslims-after-the-tablighi-jamat-event (accessed 30 May 2020).

7 The gist of the briefing on 11 April 2020 available in print can be found here: '669 са заразените с COVID-19 у нас, излекуваните са 68, Български лекарски съюз [Bulgarian Doctors Union], 12 April 2020, https://blsbg.com/bg/4412.12-april-669-sa-zarazenite-s-covid-19-u-nas-izlekuvanite-sa-68.html; and its video version is available on YouTube, uploaded by Дарик Радио / *Darik Radio* www.youtube.com/watch?v=qXA4bpyxk68 (accessed 30 May 2020).

8 See Chapter 1, endnote 13.

9 John Eligon, Audra D. S. Burch, Dionne Searcey and Richard A. Oppel Jr., 'Black Americans face alarming rates of coronavirus infection in some states', *New York Times*,

7 April 2020, www.nytimes.com/2020/04/07/us/coronavirus-race.html; Reis The-bault, Andrew Ba Tran and Vanessa Williams, 'The coronavirus is infecting and killing Black Americans at an alarmingly high rate', *Washington Post*, 7 April, www.washing tonpost.com/nation/2020/04/07/coronavirus-is-infecting-killing-black-americans-an-alarmingly-high-rate-post-analysis-shows/?arc404=true (accessed 30 May 2020).

10 Robert Booth, 'BAME groups hit harder by Covid-19 than white people, UK study suggests', *Guardian*, 7 April 2020, www.theguardian.com/world/2020/apr/07/bame-groups-hit-harder-covid-19-than-white-people-uk; Sunny Hundal, 'Why are a third of UK COVID-19 patients ethnic minority?' *Open Democracy*, 11 April 2020, www.opendemocracy.net/en/opendemocracyuk/why-are-third-uk-covid-19-patients-ethnic-minority/ (accessed 30 May 2020).

11 Melissa Healy, 'Why is the coronavirus so much more deadly for men than for women?' *Philadelphia Inquirer*, 21 March 2020, www.inquirer.com/health/coronavirus/coronavi-rus-men-boys-20200321.html (accessed 30 May 2020).

12 Silvia Sciorilli Borrelli and Matthew Karnitschnig, 'Italy's future is in German hands', *Politico*, 2 April 2020, www.politico.eu/article/coronavirus-italy-future-germany/ (accessed 30 May 2020).

13 'China sends essential coronavirus supplies to Italy', *AlJazeera*, 14 March 2020, www.aljazeera.com/news/2020/03/china-sends-essential-coronavirus-supplies-italy-200313195241031.html; 'COVID-19: China steps in to help Italy battle the virus', *DW*, 24 March 2020, www.dw.com/en/covid-19-china-steps-in-to-help-italy-battle-the-virus/a-52901560 (accessed 30 May 2020).

14 'We cannot let the cure be worse than the problem itself', 23 March 2020, 9:30 am, https://twitter.com/realDonaldTrump/status/1241935285916782593.

15 Anya van Wagtendonk, 'The government is distributing emergency Covid-19 supplies. But some states are losing out', *Vox*, 29 March 2020, www.vox.com/policy-and-politics/2020/3/29/21198704/emergency-covid-19-supplies-fema-states-federal-government; Toluse Olorunnipa, Josh Dawsey, Chelsea Janes and Isaac Stanley-Becker, 'Governors plead for medical equipment from federal stockpile plagued by shortages and confusion', *Washington Post*, 1 April 2020, www.washingtonpost.com/politics/governors-plead-for-medical-equipment-from-federal-stockpile-plagued-by-shortages-and-confusion/2020/03/31/18aadda0-728d-11ea-87da-77a8136c1a6d_story.html (accessed 30 May 2020).

16 Stephanie Mencimer, 'Peter Navarro is the worst possible person to be in charge of pan-demic supplies', *Mother Jones*, 9 April 2020, www.motherjones.com/politics/2020/04/peter-navarro-is-the-worst-possible-person-to-be-in-charge-of-pandemic-supplies/ (accessed 30 May 2020).

17 Astead W. Herndon and Jim Rutenberg, 'Wisconsin election fight heralds a national battle over virus-era voting', *New York Times*, 6 April 2020, www.nytimes.com/2020/04/06/us/politics/wisconsin-primary-voting-coronavirus.html; Natasha Korecki and Zach Montellaro, 'Wisconsin supreme court overturns governor, orders Tuesday elections to proceed', *Politico*, 6 April 2020, www.politico.com/news/2020/04/06/wisconsin-governor-orders-stop-to-in-person-voting-on-eve-of-election-168527; Eric Bradner, 'This is ridiculous': Wisconsin holds its primary election in the middle of a pan-demic', *CNN*, 7 April 2020, https://edition.cnn.com/2020/04/07/politics/wisconsin-primary-coronavirus/index.html (accessed 30 May 2020).

18 Sydney Ember, 'Bernie Sanders drops out of 2020 Democratic race for president', *New York Times*, 8 April 2020, www.nytimes.com/2020/04/08/us/politics/bernie-sanders-drops-out.html (accessed 30 April 2020).

19 Sarah Marsh, 'NHS staff making masks from snorkels amid PPE shortages', *Guardian*, 1 April 2020, www.theguardian.com/society/2020/apr/01/nhs-staff-making-masks-from-snorkels-amid-ppe-shortages; Jessica Potter, 'There are still NHS staff with-out proper PPE – their lives are at risk', *Guardian,* 3 April 2020, www.theguardian.com/commentisfree/2020/apr/03/nhs-staff-protection-doctor-ppe-coronavirus;

Dennis Campbell, 'Doctors lacking PPE "bullied" into treating Covid-19 patients', *Guardian*, 6 April, www.theguardian.com/world/2020/apr/06/nhs-doctors-lacking-ppe-bullied-into-treating-covid-19-patients; Dennis Campbell, 'Top doctor sparks anger by telling NHS staff not to waste PPE', *Guardian*, 9 April 2020, www.theguardian.com/society/2020/apr/09/top-doctor-sparks-anger-telling-nhs-staff-not-waste-ppe-prof-andrew-goddard-covid-19; 'Editorial: The Guardian view on coronavirus: As deaths mount, so do questions', *Guardian*, 10 April 2020, www.theguardian.com/commentisfree/2020/apr/10/the-guardian-view-on-coronavirus-as-deaths-mount-so-do-questions; Marina Hyde, 'With 1,000 deaths a day, our leaders should be facing far tougher questions', *Guardian*, 10 April 2020; Daniel Boffey and Robert Booth, 'UK missed three chances to join EU scheme to bulk-buy PPE', *Guardian*, 13 April 2020, www.theguardian.com/world/2020/apr/13/uk-missed-three-chances-to-join-eu-scheme-to-bulk-buy-ppe (accessed 31 May 2020).

20 'Coronavirus: Nurses demand answers on PPE supply', *BBC*, 2 April 2020, www.bbc.com/news/uk-northern-ireland-52143332; Claire Press, 'Coronavirus: The NHS workers wearing bin bags as protection', *BBC*, 5 April 2020, www.bbc.com/news/health-52145140; Donna Traynor, 'Coronavirus: District nurse voices Covid-19 PPE concerns', *BBC*, 9 April 2020, www.bbc.com/news/uk-northern-ireland-52215049 (accessed 31 May 2020).

21 See Chapter 2, endnote 8.

22 See the Wikipedia entry for TV Record, where the sale of the company to the Igreja Universal do Reino de Deus (Universal Church of the Kingdom of God) in 1989 is noted in the historical overview: https://en.wikipedia.org/wiki/RecordTV. On the Universal Church's programme linking religion, big business activity, media ownership, and championing of Bolsonaro's politics, see: Alexander Zaitchik and Christopher Lord, 'How a demon-slaying Pentecostal billionaire is ushering in a post-catholic Brazil', *New Republic*, 7 February 2020, https://newrepublic.com/article/153083/demon-slaying-pentecostal-billionaire-ushering-post-catholic-brazil; Michael Stott, 'Brazil's evangelical church preaches the Bolsonaro revolution', *Financial Times*, 16 December 2019, www.ft.com/content/e7a47196-1817-11ea-9ee4-11f260415385. On Bolsonaro's attacks on Rede Globo, see note 52 (accessed 30 May 2020).

23 'Sealing woes of residents of areas sealed in Delhi-NCR', *Outlook*, 9 April 2020, www.outlookindia.com/newsscroll/sealing-woes-of-residents-of-areas-sealed-in-delhincr/1797049 (accessed 31 May 2020).

24 'Watch: Indore mob attacks healthcare workers on COVID-19 duty', *Week*, 2 April 2020, www.theweek.in/news/india/2020/04/02/watch-indore-mob-attacks-healthcare-workers-on-covid-19-duty.html; Anurag Dwary and Chandrashekar Srinivasan, 'On camera, COVID-19 health staff attacked, chased away in Madhya Pradesh's Indore', *NDTV*, 2 April 2020, www.ndtv.com/india-news/coronavirus-lockdown-india-on-camera-health-workers-attacked-in-madhya-pradeshs-indore-2-doctors-inj-2204649; 'Mob attacks health workers in Thoothukudi', *Outlook*, 5 April 2020, www.outlookindia.com/newsscroll/mob-attacks-health-workers-in-thoothukudi/1792192; Nithya Mandyam, 'Coronavirus outbreak: Mob attacks health workers in Bengaluru', *Times of India*, 20 April 2020, https://timesofindia.indiatimes.com/city/bengaluru/coronavirus-outbreak-mob-attacks-health-workers-in-bengaluru/articleshow/75240094.cms (accessed 31 May 2020).

25 Vikas Pandey, 'Coronavirus: India doctors "spat at and attacked"', *BBC*, www.bbc.com/news/world-asia-india-52151141; Bindu Shajan Perappadan, 'Doctors seek action against assaulters', *Hindu*, 10 April 2020, www.thehindu.com/news/cities/Delhi/doctors-seek-action-against-assaulters/article31305116.ece (accessed 31 May 2020).

26 'Delhi man arrested for attacking two doctors', *Indian Express*, 9 April 2020, www.newindianexpress.com/cities/delhi/2020/apr/09/delhi-man-arrested-for-allegedly-assaulting-women-doctors-for-spreading-covid-19-2127808.html (accessed 31 May 2020).

27 'Being ostracised, asked by landlords to vacate home for treating COVID-19 patients, claim doctors', *DNA*, 24 March 2020, www.dnaindia.com/india/report-being-ostracised-asked-by-landlords-to-vacate-home-for-treating-covid-19-patients-claim-doctors-2818373; Sumati Yengkhom, 'Frontline healthcare workers face ostracization from landlords in Kolkata', *Times of India*, 25 March 2020, https://timesofindia.indiatimes.com/city/kolkata/frontline-healthcare-workers-face-ostracization-from-landlords/articleshow/74801408.cms (accessed 31 May 2020).

28 Government of NCT Delhi, Order No. F.51/DGHS/PH-IV/COVID-19/2020/prsecyhfw/3316–30, 24 March 2020, http://health.delhigovt.nic.in/wps/wcm/connect/95096c804dacdc9595abf7982ee7a5c7/oLand.pdf?MOD=AJPERES&lmod=276494546&CACHEID=95096c804dacdc9595abf7982ee7a5c7 (accessed 31 May 2020).

29 'Започна приемането на заявления за 375 лева еднократна помощ за родители', *News.bg*, 14 April 2020, https://news.bg/society/zapochna-priemaneto-na-zayavleniya-za-375-lv-ednokratna-pomosht-za-roditeli.html. The announcement itself was reported on 11 April 2020, for instance, here: 'Родители в неплатен отпуск ще получат еднократна помощ от 375 лева', *Investor.bg*, 11 April 2020, www.investor.bg/biudjet-i-finansi/333/a/roditeli-v-neplaten-otpusk-shte-poluchat-ednokratna-pomosht-ot-375-leva-302289/ (accessed 31 May 2020).

7
RELIGION

Summary: *The Covid-19 measures, social distancing and lockdown, posed a significant challenge to institutionalized religious observance. In some instances, religious institutions tried to carve an exceptional space for themselves; it was widely reported, however, that many mainstream religious institutions bent their practices to comply with the measures taken. This chapter considers how believers might understand the pandemic from a religious perspective. Theodicy naturally comes up as the conceptual area where such a perspective would be centred; some of the contradictions and scope of theodicy are considered. Interventions here move from the theological to the economic underpinnings of institutionalized religion and then to current collaborations between right-wing politics and fundamentalist religious practice.*

Suman Gupta (15 April 2020, Delhi, India)

As expected, Modi appeared on TV at 10 this morning and announced the extension of the national lockdown until 3 May. So, plenty of time for me to contemplate the weirdness of the world from my vantage point in hotspot Delhi. It is around 40 degrees C today; the ceiling fan is churning out warm air. Temperatures are rising in other ways, too. It's just been reported that in hotspot Mumbai (near Bandra station), a large crowd of daily-wage migrant workers, around a thousand persons, had gathered hoping the lockdown would end today and were enraged by Modi's announcement. They had to be 'lathicharged' – dispelled by police wielding sticks. A similar crowd reportedly went on a rampage in the city of Surat four days back. From the People's Curfew, we might be moving through the lockdown-as-preventive-treatment (a kind of curfew also, as Modi said) towards a real old-fashioned curfew to save India from the disaffected poor.

But let me mull a different theme, on a more hopeful note: it seems possible that the Covid-19 crisis has put religious institutions and devout communities on their back feet and reasserted their firm subjugation to the state and to scientific pragma-tism – though, unfortunately, without underlining their irrelevance sufficiently. For a while before the crisis, it has seemed as if various states worldwide were bend-ing over backwards to give the most freakily conservative, retrogressive, intolerant, obtuse, ignorant religious formations a vociferous and often violent public pur-chase and even real political power, alongside the relatively worldly and established state-supported religious institutions. No doubt that has always been with political opportunism and electoral calculation; nevertheless, a kind of unchecked rise of religious assertion has been in the air, with a demand that belief and faith *must* be respected and evidence and reasoning are deeply suspect. The Covid-19 lockdowns have put a check there, however transient it may prove to be.

I don't just mean that the media have loudly denounced and certain states have prosecuted some relatively marginal religious formations for messing up badly, like the Shincheonji Church and Tablighi Jamaat. In fact, I suspect those are but a tiny part of the very big picture of religious formations messing up – those are the more exposable for being marginal. I suspect that a million infringements of social distancing and lockdown measures have taken place in small to large gatherings of the faithful of all religious formations, mainstream and esoteric. I hear a few of modest scale taking place daily around me. It is not politically expedient or legally practicable to denounce and prosecute them all equally. But religious congregation is firmly pegged as a public health hazard.

Nor am I gesturing towards the condescendingly cajoling way in which leaders – UN Secretary-General António Guterres and sundry presidents, prime ministers, monarchical scions, and so on – are appealing to churches and the devout to be sensible and standoffish during Easter, Passover, Ramadan, Ram Navami, Mahavir Jayanti, Vaisakhi, and so on.

I have in mind two broader issues: the autonomy of religious institutions/repre-sentatives in the Covid-19 crisis and the possibility of a religious perspective on the crisis. The latter is a tricky one for me to consider. I do not find myself possessed of religious insights and am disinclined to be unquestioningly respectful towards unrationalizable beliefs (though I can be politely reticent). I can attempt more or less logical arguments with the shaky material at hand, which naturally gives the faithful license to be deaf to such arguments since these are lacking in . . . well, faith. Can't say that troubles me particularly.

Instead of poking the hornet's nest of trying to define religion here, I simply take institutions and formations which claim to be religious at their word.

A few thoughts from this perspective can be woven around the Wikipedia page 'Impact of the Coronavirus pandemic on religion 2019–2020'.[1]

[A digression on referring to Wikipedia: I recall how scornful my academic colleagues used to be about seeking and referring to information from Wikipedia even five or six years back – a source authored by heaven-knows-who-all-for-what-ends. Much has changed since, and far more nuanced views about the part Wikipedia plays in mediating knowledge are now out there. I am not sure whether anyone has analysed Wikipedia as a mode of *documenting the present for the present*.

An instant encyclopaedia in which multiple and ongoing editorial interventions are possible makes for a unique position in documenting present-day issues for the benefit of those following and experiencing those issues. In fact, this is quite a recent and distinctive kind of mediation. The most immediate recordings of an unfolding situation take place in the material gathered by executive agencies dealing with that situation (often confidential or publicity-like material) and those put out by the news media – the latter are our main resource unless we happen to be within relevant executives. The latter are also bewilderingly various for any single situation at hand, offering different perspectives and numerous framings. Until a few decades back, the task of setting a standard integrated record from the plethora of media reports (and executive reports, where available) rested with researchers and investigators after a suitable time lag – after careful analysis, due checks, and gatekeeping were done. Now the integration happens very quickly on Wikipedia, and a standard account – which can then be constantly modified and adjusted – is up somewhat earlier than researchers and investigators manage. Needless to say, such instantaneous integrating of diverse accounts and setting a standard account about situations while those situations unfold are apt to become important means of managing the very situations which are thus integrated and narrated on Wikipedia . . .]

The interesting thing about this Wikipedia page on the impact of coronavirus on religion is that it was put out to say nothing critical or even faintly disapproving about any religious formation. Some references to news articles on various infringements of social distancing are packed into footnotes linked to the 'Legal issues' section. In the main body of the page, there're only a few poker-faced lines about infringements reported under the 'Islam section':

> A large number of cases in Southeast Asia were tied to a large Tabligh Akbar religious event held in late February 2020. Another Tabligh Akbar event in Delhi, India contributed to a cluster of more than 900 cases nationwide. On 19 March 2020, twenty-five thousand people gathered in Bangladesh to listen to 'healing verses' from the Holy Qur'an 'to rid the country of the deadly virus'.

It is okay nowadays to be a bit uneasy about Islam in such pages; in any case, such stiffly factual points are not made about any other religion – and, in general, apart from those sentences, the Islam section is also in synch with the others. The point made in considerable detail on this page is that: *all religious formations and institutions and their leaders followed the rules, played the game, behaved like responsible adults. No one said or did anything dodgy.* All religions followed the recommendations of medical researchers and professionals (this posting seems to originate with a doctor) and abided by the rules implemented by states. This is good temperate reporting, one might think, but it is less temperate when, somewhat disjunctively, reporting this:

> Anti-Christian persecution: The government of China, which upholds a policy of state atheism, used the 2019–20 coronavirus pandemic to continue its antireligious campaigns, demolishing Xiangbaishu Church in Yixing and

removing a Christian Cross from the steeple of a church in Guiyang County. In the Shandong Province, 'officials issued guidance forbidding online preaching, a vital way for churches to reach congregants amid both persecution and the spread of the virus'.

This section of trivialities is based on two articles from those most biased of sources: Fox News and The Christian Post. These are the most censorious observations of the posting, which generally makes out that religions are nice, responsible, and accommodative formations and that bad atheists persecute nice religious people.

Obviously, then, this is a posting produced by responsible devout people (maybe a medical doctor started it off) for other devout people (the majority under lockdown) and designed to keep them responsibly devout. Let's go along with it as such. As such, it is interesting because it is quite humble about the role of religious organizations, churches, leaders, congregations – they should have and have obeyed the state. They did so without religious justification; in fact, they bent religious tenets and customs to make such obedience possible. They complied with the rule of law and scientific necessity without a religious drive by making their religious drives subject to those. Seemingly, if this Wikipedia entry is to be believed, almost universally religion has been moulded for a while by something other than religious considerations.

That makes me wonder: is there a religious perspective of the Covid-19 phenomenon? It is good that the faithful are being so obedient, but how do the faithful understand this crisis *in religious terms*? Does being faithful offer anything towards understanding the present? Here, too, the Wikipedia posting tries to be helpful. It gives a long quotation from N. T. Wright, introduced as an Anglican Bishop and an Oxford University professor (as upstanding an establishment figure as can be), which states an ideological position about religion's explanative possibilities – obviously Christian, but serving here as exemplary for Religion at large. Perhaps the person behind the posting is a Christian, possibly Anglican, along with being a medical doctor. The quotation is from an article that appeared on 29 March in *Time* magazine, entitled 'Christianity offers no answers about coronavirus. It's not supposed to'.[2] So I had a look at it. The title says it all. It argues: it's not for Christians to explain why the coronavirus outbreak has taken place but to lament it. I have seen other theological arguments of a not dissimilar sort – it's best to not try and explain what is difficult to explain if one were to maintain one's faith, one should just maintain one's faith because things are inexplicable. Ivan gave the similarly inexplicable theological problem of evil/suffering a good airing before telling Alyosha the tale of the Grand Inquisitor in Dostoevsky's *Brothers Karamazov*. Instead of explanation, Wright makes much of the comforts of lament, citing various Biblical examples of lament and some purporting to show that even God laments. Lament thus seems to be a good unto itself, an act of faith, whereas explanation is dangerously beyond faith. He forgets to tell the reader that Biblical episodes of God's lamenting sometimes have consequences. God's lament could be the explanation for a really big flood or ten plagues or a pestilence that killed

70,000 men. That aside, Wright's point is that the best understanding of this crisis from a religious perspective is no attempt at understanding.

I find that quite a satisfactory position for the faithful to take and hope the faithful will stick with it and be as obedient and responsible and subjected as the Wikipedia page – and Bishop Professor Wright – suggest when the crisis is over. And be socially distanced about it. I wonder how many of the faithful are taking this line, though. After all, there are explanations in religion if the faithful seek them: God's anger at the dominance of liberalism and rationalism, at gay marriage and pro-choice policies, at sexual freedom and racial miscegenation; the arrival of the apocalypse, the second coming, the end of days, kalyug, and so on. Freakily conservative, retrogressive, intolerant, obtuse, ignorant explanations. I bet they are out there already, those explanations. I hope science and unlocked polities will simply carelessly delete such nonsense when it crawls out after (or later on in) this crisis.

Dies iræ, dies illa	Day of wrath, the day
Solvet sæclum in favilla	Earth dissolves into ashes

(Requiem)

John Seed (15 April 2020, London, United Kingdom)

Theodicy is the specific branch of Christian thought which deals with these things. Why does God punish his faithful? The rain falls upon the just and the unjust. Bad things happen to good people. And vice versa.

It was Christian common-sense that earthquakes, floods, plagues were sent by God to punish sin, as were wars and famines. Think of Noah and the flood. But what if you were a devout worshipper? Well, your faith was being tested. Under-pinning this was a theory of history and a theory of the natural order. God's will determined the movement of history and the behaviour of the natural world.

By the 18th-century, educated bourgeois proto-liberal Christians (and Deists like Voltaire) were beginning to see God as more of a constitutional monarch than a dictator who micromanages every event and process. Instead, God created the machine. It was man's task to stick to the rules. There were convergences to utilitarianism and political economy: the invisible hand, the calculus of pains and pleasures. If you drink too much red wine and are sick and suffer a dreadful hangover, that is not God directly intervening to punish you for being a greedy pig. Rather the natural order has within it a logic. If you ferment grapes, you produce a tasty drink with health-giving properties, if taken in moderation. If you are a greedy pig, then you suffer the painful consequences. You learn by this experience and modify your behaviour to conform to the divinely ordained natural order. The market has a similar logic. Thomas Malthus (1798) combines aspects of natural order and market in his theory of population. In the big picture, it is providence that guides the affairs of man. The invisible hand of Adam Smith is taken over by Hegel and more broadly by 19th-century liberalism into notions of progress. This is the subject of the unwritten chapter or two in my book on dissenting histories:[3] how notions of providence shaped the emerging liberal philosophy of history in the later 18th century. I did a lot of research into the roots of Macaulay's *History of England* (1848). But there's also a submerged notion of providence in some versions of the Marxist theory of history.

So our own understandings of Covid-19 may still be marked by notions inherited from religion and not just for the social justice warriors now shouting about how it's all about capitalism or the paranoid nutters who listen to David Icke and see it as a plot by 'them'.

But it's a mistake, I suppose, to make generalizations about religion. Christianity or Islam are our concepts – like nations or 'races' – not social objects. They are collective fictions. We would be dubious about anybody talking about 'the French' or 'black people', and I suppose we have to be equally circumspect about 'Christians' or 'Muslims'. There are institutions like the Church of England or the Roman Catholic Church. There are doctrines and intellectual traditions. There are individual churches and mosques. There are individual people. The relations between these are always historically specific and subject to multiple mediations. I think we could find precisely the same religious stupidity among every variant of 'religion' – and I suddenly use inverted commas to question whether there is such an entity as religion. Isn't this just another Western concept which is applied to make sense of a diverse range of practices, traditions, beliefs that serve multiple functions in different places and times?

The interesting thing here is the 'sacred' and how it serves certain purposes to demarcate particular areas of life as beyond criticism and beyond the reach of the state. I remember a description of a youthful Guy Debord in a church (which may have been the Notre Dame?) leaning over a candle on the altar to light his cigarette. I was impressed! Sacrilege!

Time for some food. Another cool bright spring day in London, and the world outside my window continues as quiet as a very quiet Sunday. Interesting that material labour is the only thing that's stopped, really – all those computers and phones and forms of immaterial labour are still hard at work. And yet global capitalism is wobbling after just a few weeks of idleness.

Sebastian Schuller (15 April 2020, Munich, Germany)

I have some thoughts on religion and Covid-19.

Corona doesn't differentiate, and that's a problem for religion

A significant pandemic has been around for some time which could be tied to the 'vices' of liberalism: AIDS/HIV. For religious believers/preachers, it is not difficult at all to identify the spread of HIV with moral decline and thus read it as divine punishment for gay or extramatrimonial sex. Here contagion is constructed as contiguous with a sinful lifestyle, which results in the shaming of people with AIDS in contemporary societies, even if they seem to be secular.

This trajectory is impossible for the Covid-19 contagion. There have been attempts at linking the spread of the disease to 'vices' (I came across an article about a rabbi and a pastor who blame acceptance of LGBTQ people for the contagion)[4] – but really, it is now obvious that the virus does not care for the moral and religious proclivities of its victims: preacher and sinner may equally be infected and may or may not die. Framing the virus as a punishment due to one specific group and for particular sins is just not possible. Instead, the virus is a proper universal agent. It affects everyone, so it can only be seen as a universal and global punishment. Also, 'good' people are dying – collectively and on a mass scale. Thus, just like the Anglican clergyman you quoted, from a religious perspective we cannot but conceive of the virus as something other than an inexplicable collective punishment of a God, such that the good and holy are also punished.

This brings us to the obscure terrain of theodicy. Theodicy is a nice problem for philosophy and may present excellent subject matter for a master's thesis at a local divinity seminar, but it marks an essential scandal for organized and practised religion. I myself was raised as a Catholic. Catholicism, as practiced in reality, depends very much on the old *do ut des* of paganism: you follow the rules, you make some offerings to the highest being (or the Saints), and, in turn, you receive something.

This touches a basic logic of all religion. I feel convinced (and I think this can be supported from a psychoanalytical perspective) that we expect something from religion. On the surface, this may be a concrete blessing: I make a sacrifice to this or that deity and therefore I expect this or that outcome. On a theological level, we can add to this the expectation of some metaphysical benefit: afterlife, better karma in the next reincarnation. . . . Beneath this surface, there is a deeper structure at work, I would say. Even if a religious subject does not live in a religious society, where being zealous about God provides you with obvious and material benefits, the benefit lies in the psychological reassurance you receive. Being religious means to stabilize the discourse of the Master; the big Other is stable and identifiable, and in consequence the desires of this person are meaningful. Religion grants the subject a stable imaginary and symbolic counterweight against the shaken and disruptive world outside, which is the reason why it is still a thing at all.

Yet this potency of religion depends upon its faculty to integrate and explain reality. It must be able to frame the structures of reality within the symbolic and imaginary of the discourse of the Master, within its own fantasies in the end, to provide this sought-after stability. The subject of religion may be sure of its own subjectivity because it is reassured by the stability of religion discourse.

Theodicy is a form of disrupting this security. It basically says that we cannot be sure of God and thus not of His intention, but that we have to accept the irrational and even think, as Gottfried Leibniz (*Essais de Théodicée sur la bonté de Dieu*, 1710) argued, of the irrational as the most rational thing. Thus, theodicy is counterproductive for religion, at least within our lifeworld. At the least, it reduces the value of the commodity 'religion', which is the reason preachers – at least of successful creeds – avoid this topic. They either externalize it (if something bad happens, it's the world/the adversary that's responsible and we must resist both) or by individualizing it (if something bad happens, at the end, it is the fault of the person to whom it has happened and should be understood as a chance to return to the Divine). Thus, the irrational moment in terms of the religious rationale outlined previously is disregarded or re-rationalized.

Covid-19 now presents religion with an instance of the irrational that can neither be disregarded nor rationalized. It is in itself irrational and inexplicable, as it cannot be framed as God's Will without touching theodicy. Perhaps we could say that Covid-19 presents the discourse of religion with its Real. It is the irrational, divine, the Other that is barred by the symbolic structure of religion and yet constitutive of it; that which, if met, immediately negates the structure as a whole – as seen in the essay of the Anglican bishop cited. He cannot explain, he can only admit that his discourse has no words for Covid-19. Lamentation is all that remains, which means, in other words, that the inner economy of the discourse of religion has broken down.

Thus, Covid-19 might be expected to pose a dangerous problem for religion, as did the Black Death in its time.

Disappointing apocalypse

You ended by quoting the first lines of the Requiem. I find this perspective interesting. Religions that have millennialist expectations subscribe to the very notion of the eventual encounter with the Real, the day of judgement.

Yet, as indicated, there is a spontaneous understanding within these religions that the encounter with the Real is traumatic and may destroy religion. There are no Christians in Paradise, as there are no Communists in Communism. (The traumatic nature of the Real of the apocalypse is expressed well in Leo Perutz's *Der Meister des Jüngsten Tages*, 1923, a nice novella and a good read.) That is the reason only minoritarian sects think of the apocalypse as their present.

It is necessary for the apocalypse not to take place. Some older religions even try to actively avoid the possibility (often the reason for human sacrifices in various older religions). Whenever, like in the case of the plague, apocalyptic events really took place, the same thing occurred: the position of organized religion became unstable. First, this is because the apocalypse is always disappointing – there is no salvation; there is only suffering. Second, that's because the apocalypse is not the end. Society carried on after the plague, for instance. People did meet their end, but on the way, no angels descended from above. Nor was the throne spotted above the valley of Jossapat.

This is the situation now. The faithful may do what they want; there will be no salvation, no escape. The notion that this is a kind of apocalyptic event might crop up. Yet religion cannot use this frame to talk about the event, as this would prove self-destructive in the end. So, religion is in the complicated position to frame an event that seems apocalyptical as not-apocalyptical. Religion is really caught between a rock and a hard place (if I remember the idiom correctly).

The adversary

Historically, people reacted to the plague with pogroms against the Jews. Although this was discouraged by the Church and the State alike, people could not be stopped from attacking and killing Jewish inhabitants of cities for some years into the Black Death. The religious uncertainty and the blows to official church positions gave rise to new religious movements – like the flagellants – but also to conspiracy theories about Jews poisoning the wells.

I expect this kind of thing to happen over the next few months and years. In fact, it is taking place already. Confronted with the pandemic, people, religious or not, turn *en masse* to conspiracy theories which become their substitute religion by appointing a universal (and I think this is important) adversary who is responsible for all that. Such an adversary allows for a return to a stable symbolic order.

In pointing out this adversary, religious beliefs may or may not help, but religion will not play a significant role in this. The adversary might come to be identified with the financial elite, with the Jews (as antisemitism was on the rise already before Covid-19 hit), with the Communist-Capitalist Chinese government (which seems to be the direction many Western media are pushing). In any case, this will provide a frame that religion cannot provide.

Suman Gupta (16 April 2020, Delhi, India)

The observations on theodicy and Covid-19 spur a couple of rather wacky thoughts:

1   Theodicy is the hobbyhorse of devout philosophers. It works very uneasily with the *do ut des* in down-to-earth devotional practices and their commercial equivalent *quid pro quo*, and yet it may underpin the articles of faith within capitalism and neoliberalism. Contemplating Covid-19 and failing to discover a pattern of divine retribution for any specific sin doesn't mean that a folksy Bible-basher would be obliged to turn to the conundrums of theodicy. The Bible is, after all, an absolute text; it always has answers for all seasons. For instance, the Bible-basher may argue thus. The suffering and death unleashed by Covid-19 only seems indiscriminate because that's how God's retributions seem from below. The suffering and death are typically collateral damage in God's retributions and punishments; once you can see the core of the action, that collateral damage makes sense. So, the main protagonists are God, Moses, and the Pharaoh in Exodus 7–11, but the collateral damage of suffering and death from God's punishment falls on all the firstborn of Egypt and their parents. It's not that the firstborn and their parents were guilty or sinful, but their death and suffering nevertheless makes sense once we know where the action really is: between God, Moses, and the Pharaoh. Similarly, in Samuel 2 or

Chronicles 1, God punishes King David, but it means a pestilence that killed 70,000 people – not David, for he was punished by knowing that he had caused such a terrible thing. Those 70,000 people had not necessarily deserved to die, but it makes sense that they did once we know where the core of the action is. So the Covid-19 deaths cannot be understood as each individually deserved somehow, but as a whole, they are typical of the kind of collateral damage that God's retributions and punishments involve – to make sense of it, we just have to find the core of the action, the main protagonists of this plot. And this is a possibility to conjure with. God is not necessarily democratic; he has chosen people and not-so-chosen people – though the virus might be democratic.

2 Fine arguments like those concerning theodicy are premised on monotheism. Only if the source of justice, power, fortune, and fate are conceived as single and coherent can such a paradox appear (there's philology as well as philosophy behind it). In a polytheistic (and pantheistic) system, one distributes justice, fortune, power, and fate to different deities/spirits and works out negotiations and counterbalances between them according to contingency (e.g. if I want to get good grades in the exam, I should pray to the Goddess of Learning and the God of Good Luck and not bother with the God of War or the Goddess of Fertility). Within this logic, there's plenty of space to appoint Covid-19 as a new god, to be worshipped, given sacrifices, placated within the network of polytheistic divinities. There's a rich history of pestilence gods in polytheistic cultures – Greek Nosoi like Pestis, the Akkadian Erra, the Chinese Wenshen, the Yoruba Sopena, the Mesopotamian Nergal, the Hindu Chamunda, and so on. Perhaps a new one can be invented, Covid Devi.

John Seed (16 April 2020, London, United Kingdom)

I disagree that theodicy is the hobbyhorse of devout philosophers. It's at the core of political economy and of political ideology. Why are some rich and some poor, in national and international frameworks? Why are some paid a lot more than others? I suppose karma is another story to justify inequality and human suffering or the ways of God to man.

Paradise Lost in one great big theodicy. It was man that introduced sin and pain and suffering into this world – or, more precisely, woman. But I can't say that I ever found that account very convincing. The Book of Job is another classic literary text to investigate theodicy and makes a lot more sense. Job's comforters turn up to justify his suffering in various ways. And he quite rightly sends them all packing. It's all bollocks: there's no justification for his suffering. But when he questions God, then out of the whirlwind he is told in no uncertain terms that he knows nothing.

Sebastian Schuller (16 April 2020, Munich, Germany)

I was blindly thinking about the problem of Covid-19 from an inner-religious perspective. This is quite telling: a Catholic German literary student who is secretly still rooted in idealism seems quite likely to think of the problem of Covid-19 and religion from a religious point of view. But there's another question to be raised here. Today I chanced upon an outraged tabloid report on a radical Islamic preacher here in Germany who has received governmental subsistence.[5] He argues that his business cannot operate thanks to Covid-19 – after all, the mosques are closed and there are no donors. In other words, confronted with the state, even a preacher who is hostile to the state openly thinks of himself as a small-scale business owner, like any shopkeeper. State support for the retailing and other commercial activities of more amenable religious representatives raises no eyebrows. This should teach us that the old Marxist notion of the market as veritaserum is quite true even today.

So, religion is a market, and there are entire economic circles built upon it: from pilgrimage sites to shops for relics and sacred objects to costly rituals for all occasions.

Now, here is the thing: if it was just a matter of the Covid-19 disease, you would not have a disturbance of religions in themselves. You could go to a pestilence god or a saint of your choice, pray, donate, sacrifice, have a sandwich at the shop next door, and be happy. But, Covid-19 is not merely a disease; it is a social crisis – people are banned from doing those things. They can't consume religion at the moment. Even if preachers may find digital ways to organize the consumption of their gods, they face a severe and long-lasting shortage of customers (which is the reason churches here plead for the licence to reopen).

I would suggest that it is this economic hardship that has resulted in the prevailing theological helplessness. The faithful may still harbour their faith, but the preachers are unable to convert that faith into money. The exchangeability and exchange rate of religion as commodity is low now; new ways need to be found to keep the financial capital of religion circulating. This cannot now be done by simply advertising this or that deity or saint, as people can't pay for that by going for a pilgrimage, dropping coins in the temple donation box, and so on. Thus it is better to accept that we, the faithful, are clueless and lament the universality of God's inexplicable will. Perhaps someone will pay for that.

Suman Gupta (16 April 2020, Delhi, India)

From my point of view, religion is fundamentally grounded in social institutions. I am fairly oblivious to its affective and spiritual dimensions, which seem to occupy the devout, so let's put those aside. As such, religion in the social world is a political economic formation – naturally, all religious functioning comes with an economic rationale. (I agree, Sebastian!) This could be a barter- or market-based rationale, and it follows in step with socioeconomic development. There are two sides to this. One, religious significations (performances, services, products) are commodities which can be exchanged to grow and circulate capital. It is therefore a sector of economic and industrial activity: the religious capital sector (with religious corporations and banks). Two, religious rationality (i.e. the structure of inferences from a set of theological first principles) serves to hide religion's economic impetus while activating and structuring it. In an interesting way, then, as capitalism develops, it takes that model of rationality and, paradoxically, first disinvests it of explicit religious belief and, second, makes it nevertheless the base model of explicit economic and political reasoning. It is in this sense that John feels convinced that the kind of reasoning that is labelled theodicy also underpins modern political ideologies and economic rationality (capitalist and socialist), though they seem at odds with religious first principles and institutions. Theodicy is premised on monotheism, and modern concepts of rights, regulation, redistribution, market behaviour, and so on are also grounded in notions of unitary systems which are monotheistic in temper and follow analogous inferential methods – allowing for contradiction and uncertainty, speculation and unpredictable market movements, and acceptance of these as a solid economic reality

Seen thus, it is possible that the crisis of religion in the Covid-19 situation mirrors the crisis of the neoliberal capitalist economy in the Covid-19 situation. It is possible that the failure of maintaining religious rationality and keeping the religion economy going are analogous to the failure of maintaining market rationality and the consequent crisis of neoliberalism (the justice of the invisible hand is out, state as economic agent is stronger than ever, risk calculation and insuring against risk is defunct, etc.). This is, at any rate, a hypothesis which offers a great deal of scope for tracking the relationship between the kind of religious forces and neoliberal economic forces which have been in the dominant for a while, though the relationship between them has been obscure. It might give a clue or two about what the relationship between Trump as champion of deal-making and Evangelicals is or what the relationship between Modi the neoliberal development guru and his ultra-Hindu lobby is. Apropos of the latter – it seems to me that it is a particular point of view which takes monotheism as the basis of all modern ideology and economy, possibly a logical monotheistic *a priori* is at work there. Perhaps that pegs polytheistic reasoning as constantly pre-modern – what do you think?

John Seed (17 April 2020, London, United Kingdom)

Well, yes, Suman, I too find it most useful to bracket out the affective/spiritual dimensions and concentrate on religion as a set of social and political organizations that serve specific purposes in specific times and places. Having said that, I think I would still stick by my arguments in a *Social History* paper some years ago:[6] what underpins religious bodies is an experiential dimension, suffering and fear and confusion – Wittgenstein's point. But maybe also the experience of joy and transcendence, hence the cooperation or conflict between the religious and the aesthetic. The point being that these are human experiences that religion colonizes and turns to its own institutional purposes. This would be an interesting way into contemporary Hinduism – no doubt anthropologists have done something on the aesthetic ideology and Hinduism? Catholicism was very clever in utilizing (and colonizing) painting, architecture, music. Mr Johann Sebastian Bach, whose jingles you listen to so incessantly, was busily plying his trade in this conjunction of the aesthetic and the religious.

I say 'religion' does this, but of course it is people and organizations and interests — and there is generally conflict over where precisely hegemony lies. Religion is the form that culture or common sense takes in the absence of education and other cultural institutions. The cutting edge of the secular in 18th-century Europe were the wealthier and more educated male bourgeoisie. In the aftermath of the French Revolution, it becomes more complicated, and the powers-that-be are more cautious about secularizing the world and more instrumental in how they handle the religious sphere.

So, yes, I concur that there is no essential content to 'religion' — it is what religious institutions say it is, and that has little to do with theology or metaphysics and a great deal to do with economics and politics. Theodicy is just one potentially interesting way into the very sensitive point of how the established reality is to be legitimized in religious terms. Back to why innocent people suffer. In secularized form, it is why some people are rich and some people are poor — from divine intervention to Smith's invisible hand to Hegel's progress of the spirit to Darwinian logics of evolution. They are each, in one way or another, secularized theodicies that serve to legitimize what is, that is, *what is* as *what is right and inevitable*.

But religion is a tricky beast to manage, and it frequently runs amok. Modi, for instance, may find his Hindu supporters an unstable foundation. It depends upon the capacity of tens of thousands of Hindu preachers and intellectuals to continue to make sense of the sufferings and confusions of tens of millions of Hindu affiliates. It's a massive effort which has to continually — daily — reproduce its authority and legitimacy. Modi is, in his way, as much their follower as they are his. It may take him off in unexpected directions or may destroy him entirely.

Anyway, there's something annoying in thinking seriously about religion. An angry atheist in me fights against my rational and scholarly persona. But the latter, in turn, tends to regard the former as an unregenerate Catholic dogmatist. A Catholic atheist! But he in turn is suspicious of the rational scholar of religion as just one more liberal bourgeois Protestant, indifferent to truth and liable to tolerate the intolerable. And so they squabble and bore each other into temporary submission. Just as the religious is suffused with secular and material realities, so too the secular conceals religious discourses and institutional structures.

I seem to recall an Arthur C. Clarke story in which many different civilizations across several galaxies pool all their knowledge into one giant computer. Their first question: is there a God? And the reply: there is NOW.

Sebastian Schuller (17 April 2020, Munich, Germany)

Suman, your previous observations reminded me of a story that a friend from the Democratic Republic of Congo once told me. This friend, an artist, lives in Bukavu but occasionally visits villages in the countryside for her work. These villages are in the grip of militias (a.k.a. mercenaries paid by mining companies) and Evangelical churches. The power of these churches is immense. My friend once had a quarrel with a preacher who was so enraged that, during the following Sunday service, he announced that this friend is cursed by God and will surely die within two weeks – a prophecy tantamount to a death penalty. My friend, fearing not so much the wrath of God as of local henchmen, fled to Rwanda and stayed there for three weeks. Then she returned to this village to prove that God has 'forgiven' her, securing a symbolic victory over the preacher.

Apart from being a nice anecdote, this story tells us two things. First, the power of these churches is not much different from the power of the local militias. Not only do they organize the market for religious commodities, but in doing so they become agencies of social domination, wielding excessive if not ultimate power over the social life of these communities. Second, the rationale of the expansion of Evangelicalism imitates very closely the general rationale of mining companies and their mercenaries. What happens is this. A church from the United States wants to expand into new territories – in this case in the east of the Congo. They send missionaries, of course. These missionaries act like agents of the big mining companies: they secure the support of local elites through money, sometimes they buy off local militias, they try to replace local power structures with their power structures (e.g. children of the old elite and devout followers are sent to school with church money) until they firmly control all aspects of the community's life. When they have achieved this, unlike the mining companies, they do try to train local followers to become preachers in order to expand autonomously within this region – we could say, in a very crude comparison, that they step out of primitive accumulation and develop the local market.

I want to take this example and push it a little bit further by relating it to Evangelicalism in the United States. We can observe here, on the very surface, a logic at work that reminds me of Moishe Postone's work.[7] A basic drive of capital (religious capital that is) makes it necessary for the evangelical churches to expand. They act just like corporations in this respect. Yet this logic of expansion is not limited to an inner economic structure alone – or in our case an inner religious one. The missionaries may state (and firmly believe) that they do their work to save pagan souls; that is, they may conceive of their work only in inner-religious terms (as all missionaries/priests/preachers ever did perhaps, leaving aside cynics), just like the trading agents might think of their business as a solely economical one. But as economical/religious business, this is all about social domination. You cannot separate the work of the missionary from social domination in the Congo, and neither can we separate, as Postone told us, capital from social domination. It very much IS social domination.

So we find a parallel here that is in reality a convergence, because, as we know, the evangelical churches do not merely act as business enterprises, but they ARE business enterprises and need to expand.

But where does neoliberalism come into play?

To answer this, let's observe more closely the nature of the commodity these churches sell by still drawing upon the Congolese experience and its relation to US Evangelicalism. Just as in the Congo, though with less violence, Evangelical churches in the United States are forces of social domination. They organize the social life of their followers, usually in communities of several tens of thousands per church. Of course, these believers/clients get religious contentment; besides this, the churches offer spaces of social interaction (necessary in a country where the public sphere has vanished), spare-time activities, entertainment (we all know of Christian rock festivals), community experience, and education – well, an education of sorts. On the last, I am reminded of my visit to a 'museum' of such a church in Kansas. It was a museum of natural history, stating that it would cover the whole history of the earth. All 6,000 years (sic). If you subscribe to these churches, not only do you get an entry card to a better afterlife – in fact, I doubt that's predominantly why they have their followings – you are also integrated within a stable community. Your act of faith/consumption grants you an embedded identity in a social framework which you would otherwise lack. In the Congo, as in the United States, the main rationale of the church is to provide this framework and thereby organize social domination.

Faced with this situation, theology appears of little importance. More often than not, these churches have no established theology at all; they follow a logic that we could, with the wonderful terms we once explored, describe as 'exegetical'. The preacher claims that he (I think 80% of the time it is a 'he') has a unique understanding of the absolute text, like the Bible, and that other traditions, especially the Roman church, deviate from the absolute text by allowing interpretations, that is, by hermeneutics. The believer of the church is in consequence asked to believe the message of the preacher and to interact with the Bible itself accordingly to find the will of God in the text. In other words, if you want to be a faithful believer, you have to consume the words of the text and the message of the preacher by attending services and/or Sunday schools, and so on.

This is not so different to any religion perhaps, but the difference starts when we think this logic through from the point of view of the believer. The act of consumption is not just an external affair (it is not enough just to go to the service once a week and pray), you have to let the religion/God consume your life. You need to devote your daily routine to God, your sexual activities, your spare time, and so on. A Catholic can go and party, have sex, do more or less as she pleases, and then enter the religious sphere again and consume a religious commodity (e.g. a confession) without conflating the two realms. An Evangelical needs to integrate her life within the religious sphere; she must let her identity be consumed by the faith and constantly repeat acts of consumption of religious commodities: Christian music, Christian parties, Christian this and that, all provided by her church/community.

This consuming consumption is not alien to the market of today. In fact, in a smaller scale, the market enforces this logic. You do not just buy vegetables, for instance: you buy the organic product raised by your local farmer and thus you get a good conscience and also an identity (the metropolitan, green-eco-conscious, for instance, the vegan rebel, the metropolitan connoisseur of retro design, etc.). Oftentimes, brands are followed with religious devotion – I know at least one friend who is prepared to start a holy war over the best brand for running shoes.

And consumers extend the act of consumption; they actively participate in it: from open Toyotaism to following your preferred brand on Facebook, providing data for the company, and so on. Just as in the case of the religious commodity, your act of consumption entails in the modern market moments of being consumed.

This is due, I would claim, to the underlying logic of neoliberal ideology. Weber once described the inherent connection between Liberalism and Protestantism (*The Protestant Ethic and the Spirit of Capitalism*, 1905). As I recall, admittedly vaguely, his main point was that Protestantism encourages an inner-worldly asceticism. As an individual, you work and obey the rules, and thus you receive wealth, which is tantamount to receiving divine grace (and sign of this grace). So, at the centre of Protestant ethics, we find work – labour as labour is the object *petit a* so to speak. There is nothing to be gained through labour, but your labour is what you desire. Interestingly enough, this is the logical rationale Trump follows. I have read several of his books – and I particularly recommend *Think Big and Kick Ass*,[8] a really interesting read and well written book, which offers a better insight into Trumpism than hundreds of pages of American liberal news outlets. In all of them, he announces that his real desire is work, that he cannot think of other things than work, and he recommends this to his followers. In one of his books, he advises them to only do something they want to do, as they would never ever be successful if they did their work for an external reason.

Trump's ultra-Protestant thinking is at odds with a certain neoliberal fantasy and may be one reason (among others, like his vulgarity) for conflicts with the Evangelicals, which makes Mike Pence, his Evangelical complement, so extremely precious for him. The neoliberal fantasy (I follow Jodi Dean's argument here)[9] consists precisely of the idea that the market is able to satisfy your desires. That is, through consumption, the desires of the consumer can ultimately be met. Thus, the market is a means and not an end in itself. There are an abundance of cultural artefacts which relate the same story of people who were too excessive in their adherence to the market and therefore failed to realize their desires. Of course, we know that the market cannot satisfy the desires and so needs to cater to repeated acts of consumption over and over again . . . the discrepancy of desire engendered by the market and its ultimate inability to satisfy is the immanent lack of the market itself. And this rationale is the inner theological and practical structure of Evangelical churches. You consume to get your desires satisfied, but each act of consumption has an immanent lack. It's not enough to go to the services; you have to attend the social life. You have to consume and let your life be consumed, again and again – if you transgress, it's because you did not consume enough of the commodity. Bad thoughts, transgressive desires, and so on are nothing to confess and get rid of but signs of incomplete and incoherent consumption. A believer is homosexual? It is necessary to intensify consumption (pray more, receive treatment, etc.). A faithful person has doubts? Pray, read the Bible, get in touch with your preacher. Somebody is in difficulty? Consume, reach out to your community, and so on. The logic of consumption (and not a Protestant work ethic) is at the core of Evangelicalism and its theology. It does not prescribe and describe a god of prohibitions and sins, nor a work ethic (like Protestantism), but a religion of consumption, where you can get your personal connection with the sphere of the Divine through consumption.

This fantasy entails the idea of absolute consumption. Not only your religious devotion but your whole identity must be based on the permanent consumption of the religious commodity, which makes it necessary for your church to provide a wide range of products and services which aren't necessarily and inherently of a religious nature. And this, again, makes it necessary and possible for the church to become a force of social domination. To realize its inner potential of consumption, it must reach out and address the totality of social life.

Just like neoliberalism.

Now: Evangelicalism (and Islamism to a certain extent) seem quite capable of doing this. Yet I would not necessary want to believe that monotheism is necessary for this. As long as you have one God, you have one ultimate commodity, the super commodity, so to speak, that ultimately will be there. This logic can fail. It does fail when desires aren't satisfied, that is, when the market breaks for whatever reason. This is what happens in the face of Covid-19. An external factor presents us with something real that cannot be addressed adequately through consumption alone. Theodicy does not work, as we have established, and it especially does not work within the frame of Evangelicalism – of religious production dependent on exegetical practices. The reason is that theodicy breaks the fantasy of neoliberalism: it states that you cannot receive satisfaction through consumption, for there is an irregularity that cannot be explained. So the moment of theodicy is tantamount to stating that the inherent fantasy of religious consumption is flawed – and this is what happens in the case of neoliberalism as a whole at the moment. The structure is breaking, ideologically at the least, and it becomes obvious that the market cannot address basic needs. The unseen hand seems to have a sprained ankle somewhere . . . which renders the fantasies and thus the inner structures of the logic of capital accumulation void.

And yet, we might conceive of another neoliberal theology. If I assume that there is no ultimate commodity – ONE god – but either a plurality of godly commodities or even no god at all but something impersonal (nirvana, for instance), I could avoid the problem of theodicy. Or, in other words: if the irregularity happens, my market might not break, I can simply ascribe it to this or that god/ instance or offer commodities (e.g. practices of meditation) that might help you to cope with the situation without the need of explaining it. The irrationality, then, is not a departure from the logic of religious consumption, but the irrationality is immanent to the consumption. You know that you cannot address all desires if you are a Western Buddhist, but you accept irrationality as part of your experience and understand your religious commodity as a means to cope with this irrationality. Your desire is not ultimate satisfaction, but you consume your satisfaction at any moment immediately – it lies precisely in the knowledge that you are satisfied for the moment and that you have a technique (be it meditation, be it contact with a guru, be it access to temples) that may help you to cope with any given situation and problem individually. So this religious practice is super fluid, more spontaneous, and prepared to integrate chaos within its own logic and theology (or better, lack thereof).

We could say, perhaps, that this theology is the logic of those working within the cores of neoliberal economy, the hedge-fund managers, bankers, traders, and so on. They do not care for the market as a whole or have any faith in it but enact each situation anew, knowing that it is not the invisible hand that will save them but, in the end, the state. Thus, they are not so much like an Evangelical believer who may be inclined to consume and hope for the best, but more like the Western Buddhist, adapting to every situation as they exercise their conviction that their debts/doubts will be socialized, will become a matter of better meditation or following the advice of a guru.

This may be conceived as an authoritarian mode of neoliberalism, where the market belief is connected to the belief in the state as agent of the market. Thus, my idea would be that Hindu nationalism, for example, is not so much a sign of a belatedness of Indian society but of its advanced position. The emphasis on polytheism could be read as the dawn of a new and many-headed monster, an authoritarian neoliberalism, where market and state . . .

Milena Katsarska (17 April 2020, Plovdiv, Bulgaria)

Evangelicals on a mission in Africa and in their domestic context in the United States have often struck me as different 'on the ground', which is not necessarily an immanent difference but a contextual one – in terms of what exactly surrounds the social dominance of any one church. In the first instance, there could well be nothingness or an alternative that has to be ground to nothing by Evangelicals, while in the second instance, there's definitely the next church around the corner (the promise and the reality of it). In a way, the US Bible belt is a competitive market with a large number of corporations dedicated to catering to consumers, a plethora of Evangelical churches each growing its flock (I am looking back to a brief sojourn in Abilene TX). Evangelical churches compete on the domestic market but also in their colonial explorations/missions; having an overseas post is a marker of how big a niche one has captured in the market. They can afford, in fact, to ostracize and expel members, without necessarily pushing them toward the ultimate consumption of their product. In Abilene, for instance, within a couple of square miles, there would be one for which homosexuality is a 'deal breaker', but another one down the road can and will be more flexible. The class and wealth of a congregation's members (with their consolidated resources and the entire portfolio of services they could offer – a whole social life) will possibly play a part in this and be ostensibly different from another congregation, but not necessarily so. As competition in the market continues, it is possible for the stocks of one or the other church to rise or fall.

Knowing some people on the ground actually paints a somewhat more nuanced picture of what each consumer takes in wholeheartedly and in 'good faith'. My friend N comes to mind here from one of the lesser such churches in Abilene.

No doubts about his faith, far from a cynic, and at the same time with a sharp awareness of the boundaries and social/economic territories between his own and the next church. Curious about everything, no stranger to occasional joints or liquor, deeply grateful for everything that his church has given him. But no 'bad faith' there.

Suman Gupta (17 April 2020, Delhi, India)

Sebastian: let me offer some notes on your remarkable flight of weaving the dystopian effects of institutional religion, especially Evangelicalism, and neoliberal order. I think you have put your finger on an important pulse of our time; at the same time, there are various points in the argument on which I demur.

Trump's texts

Let me start with a matter of detail in demurring and yet a detail with not insignificant consequences in your argument: Trump's Protestant conviction in work that you infer from his books. This is based on your putting greater weight on the long text of the books bearing Trump's signature rather than on the numerous, continuous productions of short texts bearing that signature too. His millions of Twitter messages since becoming President, his briefings/interviews and speeches (which are actually disjointed accumulations of short texts – a machine-gun spatter of slogans, clichés, provocations, contradictions). The Twitter messages and interviews/speeches and so on are chaotic fluid ground. What's avowed at one moment is disavowed the next, what's said has no relation to what's known, what's known seems to become twisted into something else, total fantasy or nonsense is stated as if it were common knowledge. It is natural that a researcher would wish to privilege his books. After all, books are readable as sustained position statements. It is easier to neglect the short-text messages that are more strongly associated with Trump.

And yet there is something out of synch here. There is nothing in those short-text messages to suggest that there is a sustained position behind them. Suppose Trump didn't have those books with his authorial signature attached? Then you are like a Brazilian intellectual trying to make sense of Bolsonaro's position: a vertiginous spiral into the chaos of continuous instability and contradiction. But Trump has those books bearing his authorial signature, and yet they are out of synch with what we get from him continuously. The obvious question that arises is: did Trump *write* the books he has intellectual property on as *author*?[10] This is a difficult question. It need not be that he has simply put his name to something written by a hard-working Protestant. There might be an army of contracted and employed ghostwriters and editors (in a workaholic Protestant firm) making a story out of – massaging consistency into – a mass of contradictory, fluid, nonsensical short texts. Is Trump the author of this? Does this narrative tell us much of Trump's position? All we know is that Trump enjoys the profits that come from selling those books, and that makes him smart.

That raises another question: how to deal with the chaos of Trump's short texts? My Brazilian friend was asking this for Bolsonaro, because there are no books to look to there; the chaos of short texts is all there is. Is this chaos a new thing, should it be understood as a kind of aesthetic, a performance without content of being the anti-establishment leader? Where to start? Well, there are two handles that come to mind:

- On the one hand, they do push some consistent buttons in the midst of the chaos. The buttons they push are transparently those that have been pushed numerously before; their audiences know how to respond to these buttons, though shrouded in dog-whistle politics and the instability of constant contradiction. They press: racism, sexism, xenophobia, militarism, the version of nationalism that goes with that, the version of religion that goes with that, serving self-interest, serving the elites, financializing the public sphere, and so on. So, in the midst of all the shifting ground, the messages that get through do so because they are already embedded in some way: they are messages of the past renewed. For example, Bolsonaro echoes dictatorship-period phrases and policies constantly, and Trump echoes white supremacist phrases and associations constantly, and they all hit home, even for those who can't believe that they can be seriously doing that.
- On the other hand, the means of pushing those buttons have been recently developed: social-networking and audience-targeting technologies. The seeming chaos of the discourse is because we are focusing on the messages in themselves and expect them to reveal a structure of thinking, an ideology, a position – but this structure is not wholly, or even predominantly, *in* the messages. The structure is an underlying technostructure; it is more than ever about when and to what end and how messages are constructed and delivered at a given juncture. To understand the structure in the chaos, one needs, I think, to understand the technological structure of the communicative system through which the chaos is foregrounded.

Denominations

Another point of doubt: I have always felt sceptical of Weber's argument about the Protestant ethic and capitalism (*The Protestant Ethic and the Spirit of Capitalism*, 1905). The scepticism is thus: *if* we assume that Christian denomination is a significant social fact (almost in a Durkheimian sense), *then* we can home in on Protestant ethic, and *then* we can formulate such a hypothesis and find evidence for it. But can we make those assumptions innocently, without already privileging a religious worldview? Which is to say: industrial capitalism is an overdetermined area – there are more explanations for its outcomes, more factors for its working, than any one. We could equally go about it by looking to social relations of class, gender, geopolitical traditions, geographical resources, material conditions, historical stage of development, states of technological knowledge, and so on. If we assume any one of these as the driving factor, we can come up with a hypothesis and look for confirmatory evidence to understand the development of capitalism and capitalist social relations. So, why go for a particular religious denomination? Could that be a form of displacement in an Althusserian sense? This argument can be extended to much of your argument. Is your strong focus on Evangelicalism a displacement for the overdetermined phenomenon of neoliberal lifeworlds? Why focus on religious denominations as the structuring base? Further, is there displacement in your account of these denominations? Perhaps the peculiarities of a historical and social context decide what sort of totalizing social domination any given religious formation may exercise. At present, Evangelicalism in North America and Africa (but in different ways!) present particularly totalizing modes of social domination, but so do other religious denominations and persuasions in other contexts. In fact, I suspect that *all religious denominations and persuasions (monotheistic and polytheistic) have the tools for realizing total social domination. Moreover, ostensibly non-religious alignments, like banks and firms and military and academic units, can assume analogous tools for the same end of social domination. Such non-religious alignments may well appear to be secular capitalist (neoliberal) or socialist dispensations. But these could flip into the kind of total social domination you described, religious in means and mood. That this is in fact a tendency of the liberal state has been occasionally noted –* interestingly less a Marxist observation than an apprehension of, for instance, Wilhelm von Humboldt (in *Limits of State Action,* written in the 1790s) and variously J.S. Mill (e.g. *Representative Government,* 1851).

Consumption

Where I think your reflections hit an important pulse of our time is when you demonstrate how these tools are used to exert total social domination, exemplified predominantly with Evangelical formations and market-centred neoliberalism. The point is that an appointed arbitrary idea (such as 'There is God' and 'There is an afterlife' and 'There will be a final judgement' or, for that matter, 'markets are efficient and just'), especially when backed by an absolute text and some coterie of hermeneuticists, can be pushed and pushed to suck up social activity on an expanding scale until, gradually, it totally subsumes the view and becomes a dangerous mode of social control by some elite of the faithful. Any religious denomination and persuasion can do this with almost any set of appointed arbitrary ideas. This is because there is a common process of pushing which has been developed in institutional religion and in their counter-movements over a prolonged period – by deploying the tools of reiteration, ritualization, hierarchization, promise and consolation, community and identity, higher moral ground, victimization, control of biological functions like reproduction and mortality, and so on in the absence (or severe downgrading) of rational balance and the pleasures of interrogation and research in the public sphere. And, this too you show convincingly, non-religious political orders can adapt this equipment too, as in a total market institutional arrangement: all satisfaction here and hereafter *could* come from wealth accumulation for the purpose of deeper and greater consumption and minimization/

conditionality of public provision. It is this process of taking almost any appointed idea – picked out at whim or from displaced conviction – to structure social life around it, to build confirmatory social systems around it, to bring unquestioning obligation to bear upon it, to concentrate and intensify all explanation from it . . . which could lead into total social domination. I think you have hit the nail on the head in *showing* as much as *stating* this. In fact, your way of stating this interests me very much: your use of the word 'consumption'. It is well instrumentalized to show how totalization works; everything does become consumption with the effect of social domination for some party's benefit or will to power; at the same time, in your usage 'consumption' teeters on the brink of seeming totalistic in itself – as if 'consumption' to excess is obviously a bad thing (like gluttony or lust).

Covid totality

I have a stirring unease about the Covid-19 situation; I can't help suspecting that, having started from contingent measures, it is working steadily into a mode of religion-like social domination – in fact, Evangelical social domination focused on consumption in the way you describe it. It is because this Covid-19 order is an autonomous emergent order, which isn't emanating from an existing religious denomination/persuasion or political-economic ideological formation, that the established religions and social arrangements seem to be crumbling before it. But this emerging order is quickly acquiring the features of such religious-neoliberal social dominations. Its potential totalization of social domination can be foreseen in the way in which messages are being continuously reiterated, a morality of purity and contamination has become not so much habitual self-awareness as matters of obligatory and punitive state policing, technology to enable distancing is becoming grounded, the public sphere (news and debate, to begin with) seems unimaginable without reference to Covid-19, a constant process of deferral of relaxing control is unfolding, the possibility of indefinite quotients of control seems acceptable, a new kind of Covid-19 economy of consumption is developing, a kind of political priesthood of protecting life has emerged. . . . Looking ahead from my room in Delhi, at present I am wondering what the implications of the scientific hypothesis that up to 80% of those infected in India might be asymptomatic and therefore impervious to screening and only discoverable by random testing might be . . .

Sebastian Schuller (18 April 2020, Munich, Germany)

Somehow, days seem to pass by, and time disappears in a strange whirlpool of Corona-anxiety and a general sense of feeling unable to act. This is, at least, my experience. There is an air of anxiety and depression around this city. Everybody I talk to shares the feeling of having nothing to do and being deprived of all pastimes. I notice that lockdown makes me unproductive – which is strange. Times of lockdown and quarantine are supposed to be productive times, yet there is something unproductive in Covid-19. Maybe that could be a difference between

Covid-19 and, say, the Black Death. The latter was a societal crisis; the former is, as it hits a capitalist world, a crisis of production. Everything and everybody has halted; productivity itself seems interrupted, disturbed. Which may result in these psycho-social reactions.

But this is just a random thought. Are you able to work and produce at the moment?

Considering your answer to my points on religion, I propose to introduce a text in our discussion that I mentioned some months ago: *The Dark Enlightenment* by Nick Land (easily found as a website).[11] Now, this text is not necessarily religious, but I think it is useful to highlight several points you stressed. The text is grounded on a presumption that should be taken seriously, although it is presented in a jocular manner. There is a global conspiracy stretching over hundreds of years, from Hegel to radical Protestant denominations, that tries to realize a global, totalitarian government, called 'The cathedral': 'This is the divine providence of the ranters and levellers, elevated to a planetary teleology, and consolidated as the reign of the *Cathedral*' (Part 1). The agents of the Cathedral may not consciously know that they are enacting this dark conspiracy. It is more that they are united in universalism, since the original fabric of 'the Cathedral', its content and form, consists in universalism, which Nick Land understands as a dangerous perversion. From this, Land establishes what is for some reason called a 'neo-reactionary' theory ('neo-reactionary' is a totally misleading label, as it is clear that fascism is what Land wants). The problem of historical right-wing movements, according to Land, was that they did not correctly understand the role of the Cathedral, that is, universalism, but by themselves reproduced universalist moments (he mentions somewhere that national socialism, for instance, committed the mistake of addressing a 'people' and a 'state', thus using frames and protocols belonging to universalist thought ultimately). Thus, it is necessary to break with universalism and universalist thought to end the totalitarian quest of the Cathedral. Land's vision is to break the state and statehood by introducing small, monarchic governments, where neo-feudal overlords who have augmented their bodies through cybernetics control a populace of less worthy, biological humans. We would live in a society ruled by transhumanist kings.

There are two aspects I find interesting here for our discussion. On the one side, this easily relates to the 'Californian ideology' of Silicon Valley techies, who quite openly follow the ideals of a libertarian destruction of the state for the sake of a hypercapitalistic, transhumanist communality but also connect this political agenda with religious/esoteric beliefs in a new transcendence – the Singularity. On the other side, and this is immediately more interesting, one wonders whether this theory means that theory is impossible? Any set of theoretical/ideological conclusions that provide a conclusive and coherent programme, no matter what the content, must, if we follow Land's own consideration, end up in the totalizing fangs of 'the Cathedral', for such a programme will be a form of universalization. It will line out, even if it is ultra-fascistic, a set of total rules that can be adapted to construct a society which is the ultimate sin, as it will not break but merely reform the power of 'the Cathedral'. So, Land's own presumption leads him to a self-contradiction. He could not say what he thinks, because any assertion would render his political position unstable, as long, that is, as it remains within the boundaries of a stable, coherent text. And this is what Land, cleverly, avoids. He destabilizes his own text. He inserts popcultural allusions, small ironical interplays; he opens up new threads – like the supremacy of the white race – which are not followed through. He uses different estrangement effects (like writing AmeriK-KKa in allusion to black activists) without explaining why, even without reason, and so on. So, in consequence, his text, superficially presenting a stable and coherent object, consists of various subtexts that are only united by the author-persona Land. But there is no ultimate sense, no last coherence or frame. They are only speech acts that are accumulated and somehow assembled without the last instance of totalization.

This matches with Land's own and central thesis. In a kind of affirmative Thatcherism, the scandal is that society exists and it should be undone. The vision is of a society that does not exist and a social sphere that is only mediated through strong, ruling individuals. This vision is realized as an organizing principle in his text. Only his persona, the name that claims the *property* on the text unites and stabilizes the text (note that 'by nick land' is even mentioned in the URL of the text website), but no internal principle, no immanent totality.

In discussing the alt-right, I have always felt that what can be observed here tells us something of the communication of these new fashions and about the substance of this movement. Because I think this *is* the logic of the alt-right. There is no stable ideological text (neither as manifesto nor as virtual, ideological text) that would define this movement. It moves through short texts that are constantly produced, be it by the great leaders, like Trump, or be it anonymously on 4chan, for example. Now, it might seem that there is a difference whether the leader produces this short text or whether it is posted anonymously on an imageboard, and there is. Yet what we can see is that all these texts, as you described it, have a particularizing effect. They do not produce a coherent picture; no story is told (which is the reason it does not matter whether QAnon's anticipations of a deep anti-Trump conspiracy are fulfilled); only the symbolic act of producing them matters. Only that the constant speech, the constant transgression and particularizing, ironical destruction of universalism and its perceived agents, like political correctness, liberalism, or science, plays a role.[12] There is no discourse, so to speak, only a discursivity, a constant play and reproduction of the same patterns and transgression that characterize as a whole the right-libertarian programme of the alt-right. Ultimately, it does not matter what is said but who says it and in what form.

Now, the short texts of Trump or Bolsonaro, you mentioned, serve exactly this purpose. Their shortness consists not in the fact that they consist of few words, but shortness means here, I propose, the lack of coherence. They are not to be integrated in a longer discourse, nor do they provide a base for any coherent text or meaning. They only serve as an assertion within the moving and inconsistent movement of the alt-right, which does nonetheless present the words of the leader, to readjust itself time and again, to serve as substitute for its lack of theory and ideology.

This structure should remind us of Hegel. In the first book of the *Aesthetics* (from the lectures delivered in the 1820s), Hegel discusses romantic irony, which he overall despises. The characteristic of the romantic ironic is that he understands alienation and society as a problem and strives to realize a community without alienation. But instead of going through the unavoidable social process of sublating contradiction in order to finally understand the alienated social as the subsumption of the individual in a higher context, the romantic wants a community without society, without totalization. It wants the break-away of exclusive communities that only allow those who know the codes and engage in the ironical play of subtracting oneself from society via irony to gain entry. The ironical play is the substitute for society. Hegel used, if I remember correctly, even a religious metaphor, when he described how, through ironic play, the individual sets himself as master and god above the rest of the world, devaluating the experience of society.

From here, I would like to address the question you raised. My first point is that it is this logic of ironical romanticism that not only characterizes the alt-right but is also the principle of the . . . well, neo-religious . . . movement of the Californian ideology. The techies who believe in the Singularity, transhumanism and all that – their core beliefs are a kind of neoliberal romantic irony. They do want to become, as individuals, masters of the world and negate the value of individual life and society as a whole. It is not possible to enter their religion – for it is not a stable religion at all – but you must enter via the codes (and knowing the code means here also practically to be able to speak in computer code) and by taking part in these discourses. Only if one proves through one's actions and practice to be a worthy member can one be a member and be on the list of the faithful to be saved by the coming singularity. The knowledge of the code gives power and adds value, renders a person ultimately a worthy being. Thus, the Californian ideology is centred around the idea of strong individuality and stabilized through the actions of the individual, its knowledge and practice, as is Hegel's romantic irony and as is the alt-right movement.

Let us compare this to Evangelicalism. In many respects, we see similarities, as outlined by you. There is an emphasis on the person of the leader/preacher; there is the idea of the strong individual, and so on. Yet evangelicalism still is not an ironical community. You have, as you said yourself, a fixed text, the Bible, which is the centre of the cult, and you have the effects of universalism. I can join the cult by formally declaring my faith. This act, and not my supreme personality, or my knowledge of the codes, renders me a Christian. This is not the same and cannot, from my perspective, be brought together with the alt-right, with the constant game of transgressing its own rules. These are two distinct and different forms of textual practice.

Yet, I would admit that we see, in the case of Evangelicalism, a tendency that may date back to the late 1980s. The textual practice of exegesis of the Bible becomes more and more arbitrary. Cults like my favourite one, the theology of prosperity, emerged, and TV preachers who constantly shift their reading, adapting it to the market, appeared. The word of the Bible may still reign supreme, but it is now inserted in a constant change and exchange (for the money of the faithful), through the preacher, through exegesis, which does not follow a set of transparent rules. The opposite, what is said can be taken back the next minute, only the act of speaking the word of God is important, not what it says and how the meaning is derived. So, we see, in its most radical forms, a preacher, who just like Trump, does communicate to a denomination that is a denomination not so much because of its creed but because its creed lies in the, and here we go again, consumption of this constant practice. This might be the function of consumption, as I intended to describe it. To consume and be consumed by God, you need to personally engage with the creed. You need not only to believe that there is a God, but you need to act. Consumption means here practice and knowledge, means to know and follow codes and constantly adapt to new situations, and so on. The very act of consumption, of entering the social sphere of Evangelicals, may be more important than the creed itself, so in inversion to Weber, my approximation would be that Evangelicalism CAN be a religion without content. A Pascalian religion of mere, well, not rites but acts of consumption: kneel down and your belief has become kneeling down is my belief.

We could say, perhaps, that these forms are the forms of a religion of the market. The inconsistency, the flexibility, the constant need to adapt, to consume, mirror the structure of the market, its totalizing effect. And the emphasis on the individual, and even the idea of Social Darwinian rule – well, they correspond not only to market-enforced beliefs, but they are the reality and (in the Lacanian sense) the *Real* of capitalism. The market is not God, and it is not venerated as higher being, but the structure of religion is going to resemble the structure of the market as much as the structure of the market always has been structured like a religion.

Covid-19 may radicalize this. The resolution that the weak may and must die, the inconsistency and contingency, becomes more and more the structure of politics. We are ruled by inconsistent speech acts of different experts, through which comes through the idea that there are lives that are of less worth and should die, although this is now always necessarily part of neoliberal ideology and has become staple in discussions. This may not result in the emergence of new religions – but it may enforce and radicalize ultimately the market-mediated religions of consumption as much as it may strengthen the politics of particularization. A cornerstone of both may be the short text – in fact, Short Texts of the Discourse of Particularization (STDP). The STDP may serve as a market-based substitute for the 'ideological state apparatuses' of Althusser and stabilize new practices of ideology that allow social domination. We *may* see in the future that religion and the politics of the alt-right fuse due to the STDP. However, at the moment this hasn't yet taken place, as far as I can see. Covid-19 is a scandal for religion at the moment, and I think it will take some time until the STDPs play a role here. Yet it may ultimately come to be the case.

Notes

1 Wikipedia: The page 'Impact of the coronavirus pandemic on religion 2019–20' consulted on this date was later redirected to page titled 'Impact of the COVID-19 pandemic on religion: https://en.wikipedia.org/wiki/Impact_of_the_COVID-19_pandemic_on_religion (accessed 31 May 2020).

2 N.T. Wright, 'Christianity offers no answers about the coronavirus. It's not supposed to', *Time*, 29 March 2020, https://time.com/5808495/coronavirus-christianity/.

3 John Seed, *Dissenting Histories: Religious Division and the Politics of Memory in Eighteenth-Century England* (Edinburgh: Edinburgh University Press, 2008).

4 Rhuaridh Marr, 'Religious conservatives are blaming gay people for coronavirus', *Metro*, 12 March 2020, www.metroweekly.com/2020/03/religious-conservatives-are-blaming-gay-people-for-coronavirus/. On a similar note.

5 Matthias Lukaschewitsch, 'Berliner Hassprediger zockte 18 000 Euro Corona-Hilfe ab', *Bild*, 17 April 2020, www.bild.de/regional/berlin/berlin-aktuell/trotz-sozialleistungen-hassprediger-zockte-18000-euro-corona-hilfe-ab-70083790.bild.html (accessed 31 May 2020).

6 John Seed, ' "Secular" and "religious": Historical perspectives', *Social History*, 39:1, 2014, 3–13, DOI: 10.1080/03071022.2014.886766.

7 Moishe Postone, *Time, Labour and Social Domination* (Cambridge: Cambridge University Press, 1993).

8 Donald Trump, *Think Big and Kick Ass: In Business and in Life* (New York: HarperCollins, 2007).

9 Jodi Dean, *Democracy and Other Neoliberal Fantasies: Communicative Capitalism and Left Politics* (Durham, NC: Duke University Press, 2009).

10 See: Jane Mayer, 'Donald Trump's ghostwriter tells all', *New Yorker*, 25 June 2016, www.newyorker.com/magazine/2016/07/25/donald-trumps-ghostwriter-tells-all; Andrew Bunscombe, 'Trump boasted about writing many books – His ghostwriter says otherwise', *Independent*, 4 July 2018, www.independent.co.uk/news/world/americas/us-politics/trump-books-tweet-ghostwriter-tim-o-brien-tony-schwartz-writer-response-a8431271.html (accessed 31 May 2020).

11 Nick Land, *The Dark Enlightenment*, 2013–2017, www.thedarkenlightenment.com/the-dark-enlightenment-by-nick-land/.

12 A few days after this was written, Trump's attitude to science was underlined at the press conference where he proposed injecting yourself with disinfectants: 'Coronavirus: Outcry after Trump suggests injecting disinfectant as treatment', *BBC*, 24 April 2020, www.bbc.com/news/world-us-canada-52407177; Katie Rogers, Christine Hauser, Alan Yuhas and Maggie Haberman, 'Trump's suggestion that disinfectants could be used to treat coronavirus prompts aggressive pushback', *New York Times*, 24 April 2020, www.nytimes.com/2020/04/24/us/politics/trump-inject-disinfectant-bleach-coronavirus.html (accessed 31 May 2020).

8

EXCEPTION AND EMERGENCY

Summary: *The principles which define a state of exception and their bearing on the Covid-19 measures are raised in this chapter. The policy and legal recourses taken in some contexts by way of clarifying what an emergency means are outlined. These are traced through ambiguities and doubts but nevertheless express a will to prevent the contagion from spreading. Somewhat more worryingly, a few interventions find that in some contexts, notably in Brazil, a state of exception was marked more in the persistent undermining of emergency measures than in their regulation – where, it may be said, a political crisis superseded the health crisis to exacerbate the exceptionality of the juncture. The manner in which such a political crisis appeared and what it says about politics at large (not only within a specific context) occupies the latter part of this chapter.*

Suman Gupta (18 April 2020, Delhi, India)

In what way precisely is the Covid-19 lockdown a state of exception or an emergency? What does that mean in terms of policy or jurisprudence?

The main point about a state of exception, as Giorgio Agamben (2003)[1] sees it, is that it suspends something normal first and introduces something contingent instead. What's introduced cannot be understood without grasping what is suspended. For instance, large parts of Roman Civil Law are suspended and a Dictator is appointed to deal with the contingency of war. The exceptionality of the Dictator's prerogatives and the contingency of war only make sense given Roman Civil Law – its suspension, so to speak, fills in the meaning of the Dictatorship and the exceptional circumstances of war.

It seems common to think of emergency/exception as a substantive set of measures, consisting in doing this or that. Strictly speaking, they are only so insofar as the normality of measures (civil rights, for instance) are suspended. So, to understand the emergency measures of lockdown, the most significant points to begin from are: what measures are suspended? Milena mentioned earlier that in Bulgaria there isn't a defined law of emergency as consisting in this or that. In a legal sense, that's actually not needed – if we know what's suspended according to contingency, we also know what's being assumed for that contingency and then work out how it would be processed.

The other point Agamben pondered was the stickiness of a state of exception. It is quite difficult to re-establish the suspended normality, and the state of exception tends to become either perpetual or normalized to some degree. Of course, Agamben was working on his book as the invasion of Iraq in 2002 took place on the back of George W. Bush's 'war on terror'.

Fabio Akcelrud Durão (18 April 2020, São Carlos, São Paulo State, Brazil)

The question doesn't quite apply to Brazil. Maybe Brazil has a pervasive and continuous state of exception now, not in policy but in political practice.

It is fascinating how India and Brazil are different in their chronicles of the virus. Here the president, who was declared the worst in the world in a global opinion poll,[2] had been waging a war against his own health minister. Two days ago, this minister, Luiz Mandetta, was dismissed.[3] This was coming for a while; an interview in which he criticized Bolsonaro was the last straw.[4] He was a privatizing kind-of-doctor, with a long history of attempting to destroy the public health service, and has been absolutely incompetent in handling this crisis – but he was for social distancing and isolation. The new one, Nelson Teich, is a Bolsonarist and some kind of doctor. Every single day Bolsonaro posts or says something defending the virus, namely (1) it's not so dangerous, (2) chloroquine is all we need,[5] and (3) recently, that the contagion is already disappearing.

Bolsonaro was afraid of firing Mandetta and was losing support from the normal right-wingers. The situation had become farcical. Bolsonaro was doing everything he could to provoke Mandetta, hoping he would resign in a huff and leave without being pushed out, and Mandetta was doing everything he could to taunt Bolsonaro so that he got fired and Bolsonaro paid the political costs. So Bolsonaro fired him, and in a way Mandetta won, but Bolsonaro's supporters actually approved of the firing.[6]

Some days ago, Bolsonaro went to a bakery for breakfast, clearly defying quarantine rules.[7] I later gathered that the owner was fined for serving people – that's the president – inside the premises, which is against the law now in the capital. Today I discovered that this bakery is Mandetta's favorite. Many people are going to die because of this descent into absurdity. The news now is that the government has discovered a medicine that cures 94% of cases of Covid-19. This was officially announced by the Minister of Science and Technology.[8] Unavoidably, you cannot but see hope arising. But then you go and do a bit of research and find out that the medicine is just a vermifuge which works in vitro against the virus, but that means very little in real bodies.

Bolsonaro's tactic is an interesting one. He's going to try to control the representation of the disaster so that he can say that it wasn't so bad after all and that it could have been much worse if people hadn't followed him, and it's really so bad because some people didn't follow him. In other words, he is betting on managing to forge reality by means of the media and his followers on Twitter, and so on. He generally has a solid 30% approval rating, and he believes that if these people are vocal enough, they can give him the upper hand in the fight over representing reality. It's not unlike a Netflix series. If I were super rich and didn't care for fellow human beings, I would be enjoying myself immensely.

Ayan-Yue Gupta (18 April 2020, London, United Kingdom)

Two questions guide the following thoughts: (1) what are the chains of reasoning unique to the UK government's articulation of their response to coronavirus in their policy documents; (2) what role do these chains of reasoning play in the production of government texts about responding to coronavirus?

I am contemplating a document, *Coronavirus Bill: Summary of Impacts* (23 March),[9] with reference to the Coronavirus Bill introduced to Parliament on 19 March (it became an Act on 25 March).[10] This contains two broad chains of reasoning about two concerns: what must be done in response to Covid-19 and how to deal with the consequent break from normal government practice.

The first concern tends to use reasoning about the delegation of powers and the relaxation of existing regulations/restrictions. The general logic is as follows: given the effects coronavirus will have on those portions of society which government is responsible for, such-and-such kinds of actions need to be taken. For such actions to be taken, the distribution of powers amongst government bodies needs to be rearranged through such-and-such delegations and relaxations.

Section one of the *Summary of Impacts* ("Enhanced capacity and flexible deployment of staff") is a good example of this logic. It says: because coronavirus will lead to hospitals being flooded (meaning no capacity and not enough staff), new staff need to be registered as quickly as possible. To this end, the Coronavirus Bill grants hospital registrars the power to register anyone regulated by the Nursing and Midwifery Council or the Health and Care Professions Council into service. Concerning the relaxation of existing regulations, an example is the Bill's delaying of continuing health care assessments for people with long-term health conditions who are cared for outside hospitals. Here 'delaying' means that NHS providers can postpone carrying out these assessments. The rationale is the same as that behind the granting of new recruitment powers to registrars: coronavirus means stretched hospital capacity and not enough staff, and continuing health care assessments take up much-needed hospital room and staff. So, the chain of reasoning can be put thus: coronavirus → hospital resources stretched → delegation of new powers to registrars and suspension of continuing healthcare assessments.

Such chains of reasoning are mirrored by those of the second concern: how to deal with the suspension of normal government practice necessitated by the first concern. The point of such concern is to leave open a path back to conventional government after the coronavirus emergency is over. To keep this path open, some basic, conventional modes of government are retained. An example of this is the reasoning of the cost-benefit-risk analysis – 'we shall implement a policy if its benefits outweigh its costs/potential costs of risks' – encapsulated by those standard government genres of *impact assessments* and *risk assessments*. The publication of the previously mentioned *Summary of Impacts* is itself an example of the maintenance of some core conventional government practices. Though the full process of impact assessment under the protocols of the Better Regulation Framework is suspended for the sake of speed, the summary of impacts is nevertheless a bare-bones version of the same cost-benefit-risk chain of reasoning. The *Summary of Impacts* considers the possibility of never returning to conventional government as a risk/potential cost of the Coronavirus Bill. Hence the substance of the bill is prefaced by the following:

> policies in the Bill are designed for use temporarily in an emergency. They are strong in nature, and risks have been considered and discussed throughout this assessment. . . . safeguards have been built in to ensure that powers are only used as necessary.

Consideration of the risk of never returning to normal government is contained in the general 'narrative' structure of the summary: *statement of need and required delega-tions/relaxations* ('Rationale for intervention' and 'Other policy options considered' sections) → *consideration of risks* ('Key considerations' section). These mirror the cost-benefit-risk analysis chain of reasoning. Where the path back to conventional government is threatened by the delegation of new powers, the consideration of risk sections state the circumstances under which those new powers cannot be used. For example, the key considerations section of the part describing the new power to suspend port operations given to the Secretary of State states that the power is only to be used 'once other appropriate mitigating measures had been exhausted by Border Force' and would not have 'extraterritorial effect' on 'juxtaposed ports in France or Belgium'. The risks here are to conventional law-enforcement services – conventionally, the Border Force would have some independence from the Secretary of State.

It may be possible to summarize the transition from conventional govern-ment to emergency government as the transition from the rigid hierarchy of core government protocols (cost-benefit analysis, relation between government and law-enforcement, etc.) to a looser hierarchy. The ends of particular policies are considered too important for policy implementation to be slowed down by strict adherence to core government protocols.

The Coronavirus Act 2020 is the first step in articulating this transition. The publication of the Act triggers the publication of other documents (starting from the *Summary of Impacts* considered previously) which flesh out what the Act entails, which in turn triggers other publications fleshing out what is fleshed out in the previous round of documents . . . and so on. Searching 'coronavirus guidance' on gov.uk returns a vast array of documents detailing the implications of the new delegated powers/relaxed regulations for each sector that government is involved in (transport, local government, etc.). The number grows daily. Perhaps one can understand this cascade of document publication as a recursive process, in which each point spells out/explicates what the Coronavirus Act implies for each sector, more or less in terms of the aforementioned two types of reasoning at increasing levels of granularity. Further investigation can perhaps show how this publication cascade feeds back into itself, creating other recursive cascades which follow different chains of reasoning . . .

Some questions about this publication cascade come to mind:

1   How is it triggered? Public discussion about the government's response to coronavirus has involved a diverse range of views, from the sycophancy of the mainstream media to more outraged responses from health professionals and fringe news outlets. The cascade triggered by the current Coronavirus Act is just one line of possibility. If the herd-immunity approach had been taken, different sorts of documents following alternative chains of reasoning would have been published instead; that is, we'd be seeing a different kind of publication cascade. What made the government U-turn on its herd immunity strategy?

2   The question about the trigger is essentially a question about how government receives information. Where does it get its information about coronavirus? If the U-turn was in part due to conflicting advice from the WHO, then which bit of government is responsible for processing advice from other organizations, and how is this information passed from this part of government to all the other parts? It could also be that the U-turn was in response to a generalized backlash, in which case more or less the same question applies. Which bit of government is responsible for perceiving and processing this generalized backlash, and how is this information passed from this part of government to all other parts?

Milena Katsarska (18 April 2020, Plovdiv, Bulgaria)

My evening entertainment involved listening to a Facebook live-streamed conversation on Agamben's *State of Exception* in Bulgarian (the translation was published in 2019 by the Critique and Humanism publishers). I exchanged some remarks with a lawyer on the panel in the typed comments section. He was trying to outline a theoretical typology from Agamben while also drawing practical 'lessons' for legislation in our context. There's an array of state-of-emergency provisions scattered across legal rubrics – in public health law, in public hazards and disaster relief, and so on. In the initial days, there was a scramble to decide under which legal framework announcements should be made. Then there was the fall back on a 'state of exception' that is one step away from the only existing provision for military rule, and a law was drafted on the spot laying out the current arrangements.

I thought I could see three things going on simultaneously: (1) the 'emergency situation' which relies on facts on the ground, registers them, reacts to them; (2) a state of emergency as a regime (shifting power balances and arrangements); and (3) a 'state of exception' which, in fact, is kept as a horizon. That latter point, for instance, functions as lawmakers make draft laws with the prospect in view. My questions to that lawyer were with regard to how local or global the historical awareness is (of previous 'states of exception') when they do so. That's a topic I might pick up later with him, I think.

From a linguistic point of view, there's a bit of a mess, by the way, in how the various 'situations' and 'states' are articulated. There's no straightforward equivalence between terms in national and international contexts; there's heterospeak or total mess in terms of what is what or corresponds to what. That is to say, there are substantial slippages when I try to explain Bulgarian things in English because the correspondences are not clear and set out.

In my view, as an exceptional regime (of sorts) here, the most pronounced and worrisome thing that's been suspended is the functioning of the courts. Otherwise I don't see much to feel concerned about. But the fact that there's been hardly any litigation process for a month now is not something to take lightly, while very few people are actually talking about that. As for the suspension of individual rights, such as freedom of movement, I don't actually see these being decisively and harshly enforced. There's channelling, of course, but arguably that is within reason, not far from 'normality'. I don't see it as abrasively out there and don't see any hints (which will surely be suggested before long) of some such condition being historically embedded through the totalitarian communist regime in the recent past. But maybe I am mistaken.

Then there's employment rights: the right to work and receive a livelihood, the right to employ for an agreed wage, the right to engage in freely agreed employment contracts – these are definitely seriously affected. However, that never seems to enter heated public debate here, while it should be at the forefront. In this respect, the so-called 'national conversation' is about state support for business and compensation, not quite about the right to work. There's a reason for that. On the surface of things, that right has been differently suspended or tweaked in Bulgaria throughout for different categories of people and professions. In fact, it is only very conditionally understood as a right at all. By and large, people continue to go to work in a range of sectors (save for a week or ten days perhaps), and at the same time, there are sectors and types of employment that have just 'disappeared'. When they reappear in terms of a claim, they would be managed individually. All this completely removes the issue from the public eye.

This is not merely a matter of unionized and non-unionized sectors or cohorts of workers. It is grounded in the niches that face different approaches and regulations or even different municipal arrangements in responding to the overall general 'guideline'. I am not even sure that a decisive lockdown is discernible. Or the responsibility is (rhetorically) delegated to the 'situation', not addressed in a clear-cut decision-making process.

Besides being, as the good General described it, 'one of the most liberal lockdown regimes ever' (I tend to agree with that), it is also a regime that doesn't quite have a single decree-issuer. It's not the General himself alone, nor the prime minister only, nor is it the president; ministers for different sectors have issued different decrees that impinge upon, among other things, working rights. The Parliament has not been suspended at any moment, though there was a suspected 'contagion cluster' that made that momentarily seem possible, but it didn't happen. I can continue enumerating levels at which such dispersals of discussions and responsibilities were evident. That probably accounts for my failure to see the 'breaking away point' in what is an ongoing practice in Bulgaria.

In Bulgaria, people can go to work. Additionally, they can travel from a place of residence to a place of employment, crossing checkpoints between towns and villages. The executive power's position is that they can do so with the respective declarations provided by employers (the self-employed can issue such a declaration to him/herself). But that obviously doesn't spell an unproblematic state, for I can start enumerating clusters of work domains in which that allowance doesn't help. Say, an actor is self-employed, but where would she be going to work? Or, say you are a seamstress in a business that produces lingerie for France and your employer is at 1/10 capacity because there's no market for lingerie at present. Perhaps orders have been suspended, or there's no new one after the current was fulfilled. For this kind of situation, a 'temporary' layoff may be announced. Or, say you are self-employed relying on seasonal work at a seaside resort (that's gone). But the point here really is: which decision under what regime eroded the rights of all these categories of labour?

However, municipal authorities (at least in Plovdiv) have kept in place the whole spectrum of street cleaners, park gardeners, and so on. One might even wonder whether those haven't grown in number. I strongly doubt that's the case; it's simply that empty streets make them more visible. Other-than-essential shops have reopened hesitantly at first, as if checking the limit of the 'prescribed arrangement' (this started over a week or so ago), but these are now largely all open (no kidding). Here there's a different question – or is it? – whether they have customers in and under what conditions? Hairdressers in my neighbourhood were operating sort of 'under cover' last week, but now it is publicly okay to open them, provided hygienic/distancing measures are taken. Restaurants that were closed will continue to be closed, but there again (in Plovdiv, for instance), most offer takeaway cooked meals – who decides whether they can do this?

Perhaps Bulgaria makes for the oddest lockdown arrangement. That's probably because there is a legal mess in this respect.

Sebastian Schuller (19 April 2020, Munich, Germany)

I am writing this here at the edge of the Englischer Garten, sitting on a bench, which is technically illegal, as a 40-something woman who jogged by reminded K and me a few minutes ago (in the form of Naziesque yelling). I think this is a fitting atmosphere for some Covid-19 observations. With Ayan's notes on UK policy in mind, let me add a few German observations.

Informational policies

In an abstract way, I think we can observe the same phenomena here in Germany as in the United Kingdom. We are witnessing a crazed proliferation of regulations on Covid-19. In fact, I think it is even worse here than in the United Kingdom, due to German federalism. Every state has its own regulations; sometimes each community has additional ones (e.g. the obligation to wear masks in public), while government at all levels produces documents on a daily basis. Effectively nobody knows what is legal or not – that jogger might be right: sitting on a bench might be in fact illegal according to some new rules.

But, as Ayan noted, the effect of this abundance is a delegation of power. In fact, regulations and laws are no longer of interest; all that matters is the praxis of local authorities. For instance, the police of Munich tweeted last week that they would prosecute anybody found sitting without reason on a bench or on the lawn. They later clarified that people who want a pause may be stationary for two minutes before being obliged to move on. This triggered protests, and our local MP tweeted some days later that it is permitted to sit alone on a bench. Whether there is any regulation that clearly addresses this issue, I do not know . . . and it no longer matters. I think it is the local authorities that define the law *in situ*. (Which they did all the time anyway.)

Expertise

In this respect, there might be some differences between Germany and the United Kingdom, but I may well be mistaken. Right after Covid-19 hit us, a few weeks before the lockdown was announced, a virologist, Christian Dorsten of the Charité in Berlin, started a series of podcasts on the contagion,[11] acquiring the status of a High Priest of Corona. Shortly before the lockdown, Lothar Wieler, director of the Robert Koch Institute (RKI), started giving daily press briefings, attracting the attention not only of the media but also politicians – and became something like Germany's Corona Pope.[12] He became a kind of media star. His opinions and in consequence that of the RKI were heavily covered and became subject to daily debate. In fact, this morning K and I watched a programme in which several journalists discussed the latest statements from the RKI.

As it happens, the RKI acts as advisor for the federal government. Local governments, for conflicting reasons, have their own local institutes with their own agendas. However, the RKI is being presented as if its statements bear legal authority. And, in fact, that is now the case. As our federal government has more or less disappeared, the assertions of the RKI trigger immediate reactions from authorities. Of course, the RKI and its speakers (including this media guy) do stress that they do not make laws or propose measures, they only draw conclusions – but in reality, these conclusions are now determining the policy of the moment.

So we have entered, I would say, a strange kind of expertocracy, where the government is disappearing in an ocean of regulations, while the remaining authorities are local executive administrations and the ruling experts. All interrogations of this power are now articulated in terms of the discourse of expertise. People who protest against some state action at the moment start by declaring the informing expertise invalid, much like those conspiracy theories I was talking about earlier. But they do not negate the rule of expertise.

Fabio Akcelrud Durão (20 April 2020, São Carlos, São Paulo State, Brazil)

Bolsonaro's strategy is to bet everything on the war of narratives. So here are a few observations.

1   Yesterday's last poll showed that while 78% of the population is for the quarantine, Bolsonaro increased his approval rating by 3%, reaching 36%, which immunizes him against any attempt at impeachment.[13] His support base, however, is changing. The middle class has abandoned him, as well as a part of the elite bourgeoisie. That includes important agribusiness leaders – agribusiness relies on exports and is concerned about the damage to business arising from the (ridiculous) diplomatic tension with China. However, Bolsonaro still retains the support of big financial capital, the Evangelicals, and a growing number of poor people. This is mainly due to the US$120 that the government, after much delay and a series of technical problems, is giving per poor person. The government proposed some US$25, but Congress raised it; Bolsonaro managed to grab the laurels for this through propaganda and advertising.

2   Bolsonaro is preparing a discourse that will allow him to accuse the others no matter the outcome of the epidemic. If relatively few people die, he is going to say that the epidemic wasn't so terrible, just as he claimed from the beginning. If many people die and chaos ensues, he will either try a coup (he said so today)[14] or blame the governors for the economic downturn and social unrest.

3   In the early 1970s, during the height of the military dictatorship, there was a meningitis epidemic in Brazil, which was at first not acknowledged by the government. Statistical accounting was forbidden and news about it censored. It took three years for the government to do something then and import vaccines. Nobody knows exactly, but it is estimated that in São Paulo alone more than 20,000 people died before the disease was acknowledged. Bolsonaro

wants to do the same thing. But since he cannot just erase records, he must rely on brute assertion. For instance, his son went to Twitter to say that patients in Manaus died under PT (workers' party) doctors, who deliberately superdosed chloroquine just to discredit the government.[15]

4　The number of non-diagnosed lung-related deaths rose from 50 in all of 2019 to more than 2,000 in four months of 2020 in São Paulo.[16]

5　There were pro-Bolsonaro car-rallies throughout Brazil today. Let's see what happens tomorrow.

Suman Gupta (20 April 2020, Delhi, India)

As we know, Fabio, the prime minister here, Modi, is in many ways not unlike Bolsonaro or Trump (just seemingly more articulate), and his cohorts have been carrying out a brutal anti-leftist and anti-Muslim campaign. However, as you observed often, Modi's approach to Covid-19 has been totally unlike either Bolsonaro's or Trump's. India went into a typically sudden and sharp lockdown at an early stage. More of that later.

I was interested to note that hydroxychloroquine (HCQ) is being promoted by Bolsonaro. India is the biggest producer of HCQ (not surprising: it's a malaria drug and India has a fairly high incidence of malaria in its gigantic population), and it was in the media here that the possibility that HCQ may work against coronavirus appeared in early March – with no meaningful evidence. The Indian government promptly banned the export of HCQ. But Trump is a Modi kinda guy (and vice versa), and he has recently visited here, so he asked for the restrictions to be lifted so that the drug could be imported in the United States and naturally threw a few threats in while at it.[17] Modi complied. Shortly after that, Bolsonaro made the same request, and Bolsonaro is also a Modi kinda guy (perhaps vice versa, too), so that, too, worked out for Bolsonaro. Bolsonaro was quite clever in his approach to Modi, citing the Hindu epic *Ramayana* to court Modi's religious sensibilities.[18]

Now, the question that we are contemplating: how come Modi is behaving so differently from Trump and Bolsonaro? Both the latter have basically tried to deny it, have buckled to the extent of HCQ, have consistently tried to undermine the regional/state governments and governors, and have intermittently been leading campaigns against social distancing themselves. The duo might have the same advisors, as you observed, Fabio; only Bolsonaro is even more brazen than Trump, though it's quite difficult to be more brazen than Trump. Modi is comparatively suave in appearance, though not in fact. Clearly, in most respects, Modi sees eye to eye with Trump and Bolsonaro; they are kindred spirits, their opportunistic, ultraneoliberal worldviews gel. But Modi has become the voice of science and the saviour of the public for his followers by moving quite quickly on lockdowns and social distancing. Where's the difference? This might be where a sociological analysis can begin from.

This is a question of many dimensions. One dimension concerns the seemingly unshakable minority support of Bolsonaro and Trump. Bolsonaro doesn't want much more than a steady 30% – all he needs to keep this 30% is to be divisive. This is not much different from Trump – his wafer-thin majority and loss in the popular vote last time also delineated an unshakable minority support base, which is bolstered every time he does something divisive. The thing about Modi's support base is that it is really a majority support base – he doesn't really need to be divisive to court them. I guess there just aren't as many progressives, leftists, or even centrists in India as in Brazil and the United States. In India, those are a small, elite, and disregardable minority. Modi's thumping majority is a real representation of the electorate. When Modi allows repressive measures against leftists and Muslims, he doesn't court an adoring minority of the electorate by being outrageous, he plays to the majority of adoring voters by fulfilling their expectations – they don't divide, they unite (a majority anyway). Of late, some cracks were beginning to appear because the economy was taking a downturn (high unemployment); in that respect, Covid-19 has been a godsend for Modi. Now, this relationship that Trump and Bolsonaro have with their utterly faithful minority supporters, fostered through continuous performances of division and confrontation – this is an extremely interesting phenomenon. One way to understand the mechanics of this is to start with: who are Bolsonaro's 30%? This is a very difficult question. One guess is that this 30% comes up through a longstanding social fault line. Bolsonaro has not invented his support base but found it, and so has Trump. This support base was, in some way, waiting for Bolsonaro. Why? What is the contradiction or fissure which unites this, otherwise really quite diverse in terms of demographic characteristics, 30% for Bolsonaro?

The other side of this issue is superstructural. I have been wondering about the presidential system – where a directly elected president has powers that are almost equal to that of parliamentary bodies of elected representatives and the judiciary. That's another difference from India, which follows the British model of government being formed by a majority within parliament which then nominates a prime minister. The prime minister may be a charismatic leader of the majority (like Modi), but he is not elected as such (Modi has come the closest to being seen as such since Nehru). Ultimately, he is no more than an office holder for a party in government and answerable to parliament; he has no mandate separate from the parliamentary representation. He can't really appeal to the people against parliament; he has to carry a majority in parliament. At best he can try a kind of *autogolpe*, but that will simply be on the calculation of getting a better parliamentary majority. The presidential system amazes me – the kind of power allowed the US or Brazilian president is quite extraordinary, as if the Constitution and the relevant laws were written on the assumption that there would always be sensible polite leaders who would be conscientiously guided by good practice codes rather than hard rules. Trump and Bolsonaro are testing the limits of their office because this office does in fact grant extraordinary power to one person, the sort of concentration that may actually undermine democratic representation. And yet they seem to concentrate their power by a mandate, so actually by manoeuvring a crude formally democratic procedure – populist democracy, in which all that matters is a working majority of the demos. That allows them to undercut all institutional and constitutional guarantees of functional democracy and democratic practice. (Democracy is a much-misunderstood term and has acquired an unfortunate moral connotation – it has simply turned into moral claims on behalf of working majority rule, which is *not* democracy.) The reason systems of absolute rulers disappeared from various parts of the world was at least to some extent because of the lessons of history: there's always the possibility of a lunatic or an utterly small-minded self-centred idiot ascending the throne legitimately. And yet the presidential system has allowed precisely something of what the abrogation of all-powerful monarchies was meant to remove. In brief, there's a rich vein of liberal arguments on presidential systems which could inform a sociological analysis of the current situation in Brazil . . . and the United States, Turkey, and so on – and perhaps in India, too, in due course, if Modi, like Erdogan, can but manoeuvre it.

Milena Katsarska (21 April 2020, Plovdiv, Bulgaria)

I am not sure I would have phrased the matter of the presidential system as 'superstructural' merely because that is embedded in government arrangements that invest a presidential institution and a single person with extraordinary powers. As worrisome as that arrangement is, which should in fact be interrogated and possibly dismantled, I find myself way more worried by the increasingly rhetorical way in which the other arrangement is shifting – that of the legislative body's majority choice of prime minister. The appearance therein of charismatic all-powerful fathers of the nation is the more dangerous because it is against the grain of that system. Somehow I fail to see mothers of the nation appearing in quite that way. Boyko Borisov is a case in point, as is Narendra Modi. Unexpectedly – or perhaps quite predictably – the United Kingdom, too, seems to be but a step away from that direction or maybe already there in the form of Boris Johnson. If this structural arrangement is leading towards consolidation of the model of presidential systems, then we are all in big trouble.

Crises have historically been met by the emergence of a strong figure to rule and for the dominant majority to identify with. The current drift towards presidential-like arrangements may have something to do with the perpetuation of crises (economic and political) in recent history. But it is probably more than that. It might equally have something to do with whom the example to follow is or whom the exporter of the universal (so-called democratic) model is and how it is replicated on the ground in different contexts. If I turn to one of my favourite grid metaphors: there's a horizontal and a vertical axis here. One stems from the historical contextualization in any given nation-state context, but the other draws upon echoes and influences and replications across contexts, which are also of course historically grounded.

Saw a good point made earlier in the news about the 1 billion 'foreign investment' that Bulgaria 'gets' annually by adding up: (1) the difference between the living standards in the EU and the lower standard in Bulgaria and (2) traditional familial support ties that encourage Bulgarians living and working abroad to send money 'back home'. The latter is diminishing to naught in the current situation, taking into account Bulgarians who have returned as of March and the manner in which many of them make an income. The repercussions of this are quite serious for this tiny and not particularly thriving economy.

Suman Gupta (21 April 2020, Delhi, India)

In political reasoning, it is taken for granted that an elected representative (as within representative democracy) is a person representing the interests of a constituency. This elected person is in him/herself a transparent person, a conduit who is able to channel the needs and desires of the people he/she represents. Such representativeness is demonstrated by the elected person in reflecting the needs of people represented, as a faithful mirror, and by acting for them, as an extension of their minds and hands.

In political aesthetics, however, a representative (also as in representative democracy) is a person who appeals sufficiently to a constituency to become electable. This appeal is not so much the promise of working for this constituency's interests but much more the ability to hold their interest: through the appeal of charisma, entertainment value, dramatic verve, rhetorical style, performance skills, stereotyped image of the bossman or bosswoman (military/lawyer, white/black, male/female, etc.). This elected person is not in principle transparent and therefore a channel of the people represented; on the contrary, this elected person is so loudly opaque that the putatively represented people can't stop looking at him/her – can't stop talking about him/her, whether admiringly or complainingly, hopefully or with despair.

The problem might be that we are constantly getting these two kinds of representativeness mixed up or are talking at cross-purposes between these two kinds of representativeness.

Notes

1 Giorgio Agamben, *State of Exception*, trans. Kevin Attell (Chicago: University of Chicago Press, 2005 [2003]).
2 'Leaders risk lives by minimizing the coronavirus. Bolsonaro is the worst', *Washington Post,* 14 April 2020, www.washingtonpost.com/opinions/global-opinions/jair-bolsonaro-risks-lives-by-minimizing-the-coronavirus-pandemic/2020/04/13/6356a9be-7da6-11ea-9040-68981f488eed_story.html (accessed 31 May 2020).
3 Marina Lopes, 'Brazil's Bolsonaro fires health minister Mandetta after differences over coronavirus response', *Washington Post*, 16 April 2020, www.washingtonpost.com/world/the_americas/coronavirus-brazil-bolsonaro-luiz-henrique-mandetta-health-minister/2020/04/16/c143a8b0-7fe0-11ea-84c2-0792d8591911_story.html;   Julia Chaib and Gustavo Uribe, 'Bolsonaro fires Mandetta and announces Nelson Teich as minister of health', *Folha de S.Paulo*, 17 April 2020, https://www1.folha.uol.com.br/internacional/en/brazil/2020/04/bolsonaro-fires-mandetta-and-announces-nelson-teich-as-minister-of-health.shtml (accessed 31 May 2020).

4 'Exclusivo: "brasileiro não sabe se escuta o ministro ou o presidente", diz Mandetta', *Globo G1*, 12 April 2020, https://g1.globo.com/fantastico/noticia/2020/04/12/maio-e-junho-serao-os-meses-mais-duros-afirma-mandetta-em-entrevista-exclusiva-ao-fantastico.ghtml (accessed 1 June 2020).

5 'Bolsonaro defends chloroquine and resumes clash with governors and mayors in televised speech', *Folha de S.Paulo*, 9 April 2020, https://www1.folha.uol.com.br/internacional/en/brazil/2020/04/bolsonaro-defends-chloroquine-and-resumes-clash-with-governors-and-mayors-in-televised-speech.shtml (accessed1 June 2020).

6 Though large numbers disapproved of Mandetta's dismissal, Bolsonaro's approval ratings went up; see: 'Para 64%, Bolsonaro "agiu mal" ao demitir Mandetta, diz Datafolha', *Globo G1,* 17 April 2020, https://g1.globo.com/politica/noticia/2020/04/17/para-64percent-bolsonaro-agiu-mal-ao-demitir-mandetta-diz-datafolha.ghtml (accessed 1 June 2020).

7 In English, the bakery event and the background briefly outlined here was reported later: Jonathan Wheatley and Andres Schipani, 'Bolsonaro, Brazil and the coronavirus crisis in emerging markets', *Financial Times*, 19 April 2020, www.ft.com/content/3d113fba-8096-11ea-82f6-150830b3b99a (accessed 31 May 2020).

8 'Remédio com 94% de eficácia contra a COVID-19 será testado no Brasil', 15 April 2020, www.youtube.com/watch?v=TgPKtIGNCO4 (accessed 31 May 2020).

9 Department of Health and Social Care, UK Government, 'Coronavirus bill: Summary of impacts', 2020, www.gov.uk/government/publications/coronavirus-bill-summary-of-impacts/coronavirus-bill-summary-of-impacts?fbclid=IwAR1fLDWGg8BYa6mteM uoJVOSLVbyaiDtCYFGl8ruzbeGK-7ziQZlhGadkY4#section-3 – containingslowing-the-virus (accessed 31 May 2020).

10 Coronavirus Act 2020, www.legislation.gov.uk/ukpga/2020/7/contents/enacted.

11 The first podcast of the series *Das Coronavirus-Update mit Christian Drosten* was on 26 February 2020. All are found at www.ndr.de/nachrichten/info/podcast4684_page-4.html (accessed 31 May 2020).

12 For a video of Wieler's press briefing shortly after the lockdown started, see www.youtube.com/watch?v=9olJC_JZj-s. For an account of the growing prominence of the RKI during this period written after this intervention, see: 'Coronavirus: What is Germany's Robert Koch Institute?' *DW*, 13 May 2020, www.dw.com/en/coronavirus-what-is-germanys-robert-koch-institute/a-53416437 (accessed 31 May 2020).

13 '64% avaliam que Bolsonaro agiu mal ao demitir Mandetta', *Datafolha*, 18 April 2020, http://datafolha.folha.uol.com.br/opiniaopublica/2020/04/1988673-64-avaliam-que-bolsonaro-agiu-mal-ao-demitir-mandetta.shtml (accessed 1 June 2020).

14 'Bolsonaro ameaça democracia, discursa em ato por AI-5 e dispara: "chega de patifaria e velha política, agora é o povo no poder"', *Brasília,* 19 April 2020, www.brasil247.com/regionais/brasilia/bolsonaro-ameaca-democracia-discursa-em-ato-por-ai-5-e-dispara-chega-de-patifaria-e-velha-politica-agora-e-o-povo-no-poder(accessed1June 2020).

15 Eduardo Bolsonaro's Twitter post of 17 April said: 'Estudo clínico realizado em Manaus pra desqualificar a cloroquina causou 11 MORTES após pacientes receberem doses muito fora do padrão. / Este absurdo deve ser investigado imediatamente. / Os respon sáveis são do PT. Mas isso é pura coincidência, claro . . . ' https://twitter.com/bolsona rosp/status/1251132537373630469?lang=en (accessed 1 June 2020).

16 Felipe Grandin and Patrícia Figueiredo, 'Em três semanas, São Paulo tem mais inter nações por síndromes respiratórias que em todo o ano de 2019', *Globo*, 14 April 2020, https://g1.globo.com/sp/sao-paulo/noticia/2020/04/14/em-tres-semanas-sao-paulo-tem-mais-internacoes-por-sindromes-respiratorias-que-em-todo-o-ano-de-2019.ghtml; 'Casos de coronavírus e número de mortes no Brasil em 19 de abril', *Globo*, 19 April 2020, https://g1.globo.com/bemestar/coronavirus/noticia/2020/04/19/casos-de-coronavirus-e-numero-de-mortes-no-brasil-em-19-de-abril.ghtml (accessed 31 May 2020).

17 'Hydroxychloroquine: The unproven "corona drug" Trump is threatening India for', *BBC,* 7 April 2020, www.bbc.com/news/world-asia-india-52180660 (accessed 1 June 2020).

18 'Brazilian president invokes Ramayana while seeking hydroxychloroquine from India', *Hindu*, 9 April 2020, www.thehindu.com/news/international/brazilian-prez-invokes-ramayana-while-seeking-hydroxychloroquine-from-india/article31295486.ece (accessed 1 June 2020).

9
REAL AND DIGITAL SPACE

Summary: *The initial interventions consider what effect the lockdown and social distancing measures have on our sense of physical space. Physical space is considered at various levels: personal space, domestic space, work space, social-network space, public space. Alterations in these notions of space naturally raise significant legal and policy questions. The growing dependence on digital space – regarded here as a sort of 'mental' space – comes up, too. Various apps to trace contact between persons so as to prevent the contagion spreading are noted and their potential functions beyond fighting Covid-19 considered. Ultimately, of course, space is predominantly traversed and grasped in our regular activities, so everyday life perceptions come up relevantly in some of the interventions.*

Suman Gupta (21 April 2020, Delhi, India)

All those contributing to this journal have a room of their own (usually more than a room) and live in generally salubrious areas of cities/towns. It's a privilege we are the more acutely aware of in the midst of the Covid-19 lockdowns; it's neverthe-less a privilege which is less than the privilege of leaving these rooms with a care-free step whenever we wish. Irrespective of how liberally or harshly the lockdowns are implemented, simply by announcing them, by the authorities keeping an eye on compliance with them, by all of us keeping an eye on each other's adherence to them, by the public reiteration of the rules of lockdown *ad nauseam ad nauseam ad nauseam* . . . something happens to our relationship with the space we occupy and move within, which is also, of course, something happening to our relation-ship with the spaces others move within. There is a peculiar Covid-19 collective sense of space with regard to self and others in the making, perhaps already settled by now.

Let me mark some of the obvious features of this collective Covid-19 sense of space.

1 Let's start at the most immediate conception of space: *personal space* – a kind of invisible spatial pod around the self which is habitually extended and loosely recognized. It bears upon relationships with others: the entry of another into this spatial pod is either intimacy or violation; proximity which works around the pod covers most everyday interactions with friends, acquaintances, and so on. The idea of personal space has enough of a popular purchase to be recognized promptly. In the Covid-19 situation, this personal space seems to harden with objective measurement and the force of a rule, at a radius of 1 metre around the self, the space for social distancing. Of course, this hardening of personal space has nothing to do with relationships. This social-distancing pod around the self is a sort of invisible shield against contagion. However, once set, it becomes inseparable from our usual sense of personal space – and raises it to a painful awareness.

2 At the broadest level, the presence of the contagion is spatially conceived. It is *out* there gradually capturing space (family to locality to city to country to continents), its increasingly pervasive presence accentuating the specificity of my immediate space *in* here, in my personal space if I am outside (to the extent of 1 metre all around me), or in the *enclosed space* of home (walls all around me). My enclosed space is either keeping it out or being invaded.

3 The presence and expansion of the contagion out there are not as an ether or miasma but as a spatial network. This network traces the lines of existing *social-life networks*; it works through them – through our movements on routes between retail outlets, work spaces, meeting points of friends/relatives, leisure spots. The contagion shadows the spatial network of social life. It concentrates in spaces were social life is concentrated (shops, theatres, auditoriums, conference centres, public transport, open-plan offices – open-plan offices were a really bad idea); it moves through contact points wherever the spaces of our social-life networks offer them.

4 The idea of home as an enclosed space in the Covid-19 crisis, the only frontier after that of personal space, where the contagion may be checked or contained (by quarantine), puts pressure upon various received conceptions of this space. In one aspect, it leads to an intensification of the bind between home as enclosed space and personal or *interpersonal space*. For the solitary – especially the elderly – this intensification is expressed as loneliness and boredom (more alcohol, more computer games, more mindless TV). Where cohabitation is in question, it often leads to increased friction (domestic violence and killings have escalated worldwide) or increased intimacy (more sex? more talk? more silent communion? more carefully separated togetherness?). For the relatively privileged – those with rooms of their own – images of congested localities, with four or six persons to a room, no backyards and gardens, dark narrow lanes, and so on appear as a spatial nightmare which exacerbates the dread of

Covid-19. Since an element of the preventive treatment is tracking contact points from a given case of infection, the pressures of congestion are a clearly visualizable challenge. On the other side of congestion, the condition of not having a home, an enclosed space, as for the homeless, also arouses the dread of exposure to the virus, with no protection apart from the invisible and constantly vulnerable personal space.

5   The idea of home is also modified with respect to some of its conventional counterparts. So, for instance, the distinction between the space of home and the *work space* (office, factory, shop floor, building site, farm, etc.) seems to be in abeyance, suspended awhile. Of course, a certain number of white-collar workers had already had this distinction erased under the guise of 'working from home' or 'flexible work' – the economic rationale of that is well known. But that is still a relatively small number. The distinctions between home and workplace, leisure and labour, family and colleagues, domestic and official/formal are still powerfully ensconced in social habits – and productive necessity.

6   In another aspect, the idea of home as a private space is also modified in terms of its distinction from the *commons or public space* (roads, parks, squares, etc.). Under conditions of lockdown, or strongly enjoined self-isolation, there's a feeling of the loss of the commons. The only space of relative freedom, but a severely curtailed freedom, is the home, and the commons cease to be quite the commons because going out is a kind of trespassing – it needs a reason, it is under observation, it is a precious interlude, it involves crossing a boundary into danger and relative desolation. The loss of the commons is in roughly the same measure as the freedom of being at home is a curtailed freedom; it is necessary to have the freedom of the commons to have the freedom of home.

7   To compensate for the slipping counterpoints to the enclosed space at home, some (those with good enough access) collectively construct a virtual space – the *digital space*. The digital space could be thought of as a *mental space*. Its spatial attributes are conferred from various linked-up portals by users. This space is composed of projections of users' spaces for work, spaces for leisure, spaces for conversation, spaces for keeping books and records, spaces for traipsing in the gallery, going to a restaurant, talking a walk in the commons, meeting friends, watching a show, and so on. The spatial aspect of this is not, so to speak, *in* the technology; it is in the users' collective activity and its imagined architecture and contours.

These modifications in our collective sense of space – in those seven observations – call for some analytical clarification. What do these portend? The two most influential approaches to theorizing space might be expected to offer insights: starting either from Edward T. Hall's *The Hidden Dimension* (1966)[1] or from Henri Lefebvre's *The Production of Space* (1991 [1974]).[2] However, for the specific focus on the Covid-19 crisis, both offer a limited analytical foothold. Hall's formulations of personal space and social distance (what he calls the study of 'proxemics') build mainly upon inborn proclivities which are not specific as to context. These formulations therefore look, so to speak, to the unconscious of human communication, where spatiality is structured through the cognitive apparatus, biological adaptations, collective behaviours, and where such spatiality is represented in styles of linguistic expression, architecture, city planning, and so on. This seemingly carefully observed empirical basis is, however, undercut by the implausible assumption that cultures are monolithically mapped to nation-states – that it makes sense to speak of French, German, English, Arab, Japanese, and so on as each one distinctive and coherent kind of culture. So, there's unthinking political simplification here, or an effective depoliticization of the very concept of nation (which is itself a political move, too). Hall's thoughtlessness in this regard seems to have seeped into those developing his approach (interestingly, for instance, in Sorokowska et al., 2017,[3] which also usefully summarizes Hall-inspired later researches). Lefebvre's, by contrast, is a politically searching, questioning, and sophisticated approach to the concept of space. And yet, its great ambition renders it difficult to pin down for our purposes. His attempt to formulate a unitary theory of social, mental, and physical space such that the mechanics of capitalist production is clarified – at the juncture of both taking up and producing space – is so BIG a project that it leaves no scope for small foci, like specific situations or concrete experiences. Those can only be fleetingly suggested without pause or expansion, in a great swathe of abstractions.

It seems to me that there's a line to be drawn between these approaches. This line should neither be inattentive to empirically grounded spatial concepts nor politically simplistic/unthinking and should bear upon specific, concrete situations.

With that in mind, by way of foregrounding the political resonances of these seven observations, I pose some questions about each of them. The questions ask how the conceptions of space in those observations relate to notions of ownership; that is, how is (personal and interpersonal) space related to (private and public) property in the Covid-19 context? So, seven corresponding sets of questions follow:

1   Self-possession has been a central tenet of liberal/socialist political philosophy – in Hegel's master-slave argument, in arguments about the limits and prerogatives of the state, and in arguments for the right to private property. Could the objectification of personal space within a measured ambit (1 meter around) be regarded as a strengthening or weakening of self-possession?

2   The enclosed space of the home is formally (legally) conceived as being private, either by ownership (private property) or by occupation (private habitation), with a strong bias toward the former. Ownership has repeatedly and legitimately superseded occupation; rights by habitation are usually conditional to ownership. Does the current emphasis on the enclosed space to keep out (by isolation) or keep in (by quarantine) the contagion be seen, even for a transient period, as shifting the emphasis in favour of occupation over ownership? Does

the tenant get the upper hand over the landlord in the Covid-19 interregnum, at least in principle?

3　Does the mirroring of the passage of the contagion along the existing matrix of social-life networks inevitably mean that preventive treatment will up the stakes of surveillance and policing of those networks? Should the social-life networks themselves be regarded as infected, such that the medical recourse for the authorities is an invasive procedure on those social-life networks themselves (of tracking, shutting down, observing, purifying and sanitizing, etc.)? How will we know when the infection is gone from the social-life networks?

4　Can the intensification of personal and interpersonal life in the enclosed space of the home under Covid-19 conditions be regarded as a sharpening of property conflicts within this space? Where there is domestic abuse, it may well involve gendered or patriarchal possessiveness. A heightened dread of congested space must bring to mind the dispossession that usually produces such a space. Heightened conflicts of ownership and dispossession seem to radiate out of the locked-down environment.

5　Where the counterpoint of work and home is erased, would it be correct to think that employers are getting a foothold on workers' homes – are, to some extent, making a proprietorial move into workers' homes?

6　Could the sense of loss of the commons under the Covid-19 lockdowns be considered a loss of public ownership? Have state ownership and public ownership been effectively delinked so that state ownership behaves as private proprietorship and public access becomes a privilege rather than a right?

7　Who owns the mental space that is the digital space, and on what terms? Is this space owned in the way land or houses are (with boundaries and walls, etc.), or is the mechanics of ownership different? Perhaps we can argue that owning a platform is ownership of a bit of the digital space, or having intellectual property claims of some digital capacity is effectively ownership of some digital space. However, since the digital space is a mental space – is it reasonable that owning a digital tool becomes the means of owning some of this collective mental space?

Milena Katsarska (21 April 2020, Plovdiv, Bulgaria)

Let me consider some of these questions by turn.

1　For the consolidation of that personal bubble as an ownership claim, we would probably need some sort of personal litigation, that is, a lawsuit brought by Citizen X against Citizen Y for not respecting her personal bubble. Such an ownership claim can be understood in terms of analogous areas: (1) currently defined violations of property (burglary, damage, trespassing) and of bodies (rape, aggravated assault); (2) third-party regulation of spatial norms, as in any recognized authority allocating a spot within a shared space (for busking, for parking, etc.); (3) invasive behaviour which does not necessarily involve contact (such as stalking, invasion of privacy by spying). Each of these became legally actionable at particular historical junctures, and each thereafter introduced clarifications of nuances and regimes for policing, monitoring, and prosecuting. But none of them quite covers this specific kind of concretization of the personal space by social distancing norms, though all of them could be useful for giving it legal definition. Once defined and legislated on, this concretization could slip away from exceptional contingency to a standard system.

2 This surprised me – it hadn't occurred to me to make the distinction between ownership and occupancy as possibly conflicting. How can we know whether the Covid-19 situation has worked to favour occupancy? The laws have not changed. In this case, I think, the vested interests built upon ownership are so embedded in legal, economic, and cultural terms that any favouring of occupancy will only be temporary. Landlords may be currently under some kind of injunction not to evict tenants for, to take an example, non-payment of rents because that would amount to endangering the life of the tenant. I suspect that in this instance, nothing more will happen; the landlord will just have to be patient and before long will have all her usual prerogatives restored. But it is worth considering the balance of occupancy and ownership of lived-in property in law – now that squatter rights seem increasingly anti-social and tenancy rights are constantly eroded. Maybe the prolongation of lockdown will raise the issue. Since we are now into the second month, that could be considered substantial enough time to undermine standard contracts which usually provide for a one-month notice. Here employment will enter the picture too, for loss of income has an unarguable relationship to paying rent.

3 This is a very tricky question. There's little evidence that the contagion will be gone from social-life networks, literally. So far people are asked to give, and they voluntarily give some information on their social-life networks, for the sake of effective medical monitoring and counter measures. There's clear evidence that people also withhold information at the same time. There's a slippery slope there. There's at least 20 years now of intensive tracking of social contact networks as a kind of 'political contagion' of terrorism, since 9/11. There's a considerably longer history of such tracking for various areas of criminal activity. Perhaps the tracking and regulating of this current allegedly apolitical contagion could define new kinds of crimes and criminalizations of human activity. One should keep a close watch on this.

5 On the point about workspace encroaching into home space: that issue is in the air already, as 'working from home' arrangements have been increasingly firmly pushed in various employment sectors. I hope that the Covid-19 situation will actually put this into relief and raise some necessary legal and policy questions about 'working from home' stipulations in general. I feel very uneasy about the upbeat spirit with which pre-Covid 19 'working from home' is cited to normalize extraordinary arrangements made to temporarily shift work online where possible. On the one hand, the argument goes that

those 'working from home' people's arrangements are so flexible and orderly that they are unfazed by this crisis (no pressure on their employment). On the other hand, different types of jobs are now being understood as transferable to home with slight modifications or miniscule investments. The contractual nuances, distribution of responsibilities, qualitative/quantitative losses in both work experience and production that is being entailed have occasioned negligible discussion.

6   The issue about loss of the commons is also troubling me big time. Yet in this, too – now that we are in the second month of lockdown – we can observe an accentuation of previously existing practices (rather than arrangements). For interblock spaces in Plovdiv, for instance, where maintenance is definitely the responsibility of municipal authorities, neglect is more common than not. This has been so much so that occasionally local communities step in and invest in maintenance themselves (the courtyard next to my block is a case in point) and then get slapped on the wrist by municipal authorities if they get 'too creative' or are perceived as taking possession. At the same time, the access to big flashy commons maintained solely, as well as owned, by municipal authorities, to which, however, every single local-taxpayer contributes, was cut off in a jiffy from those taxpayers – for a month already. That goes for parks and hills, not to mention all the galleries and municipal culture centres, and so on. Currently, it is that small-scale neglected niche of interblock spaces that is functioning as commons, not only for the immediate inhabitants of the two blocks but also for anybody who comes in from the vicinity.

Talking of the commons: my evening walk to old town and back yesterday was quite fun, as the streets were again spectacularly devoid of idlers. The amusing thing was that in roaming about, I met at least eight or ten small family-like or individual parties who were all acquaintances or friends. There's no such thing as a totally solitary walk here, really, at least not in the centre of Plovdiv, and not for someone who's been living here for close to 50 years. The physical exercise was crowned by watering the block garden (one of those interblock spaces) with buckets, which is how I struck up a better acquaintance with two people from the block opposite. They turned up to give me a hand, and we discussed possible measures for not allowing the space to be taken over by parked cars once all restrictions are lifted. One, a technician, said he could assist in getting to the water tap in the middle of the yard, which is currently buried under a lot of debris. The latter pointed out that this might be illegal from the point of view of municipal authorities. But none of us felt particularly worried about it at this time.

Suman Gupta (22 April 2020, Delhi, India)

I have been thinking about apps to combat Covid-19. Google and Apple have partnered to produce one to combat the threat of contagion as a public-spirited move, as a demonstration of corporate responsibility, the Trace Together app. As

I understand it, this is a way of tracking contact points between devices. The movements of mobile devices (and so their owners) can be and are tracked constantly; for those who have uploaded this app, it is possible to track when two devices are close enough for the virus to be passed from one to the other. When one such person is reported or self-reports being infected, a message goes to all persons who have the app and have been within the critical distance to the infected person within a critical period – with advice on self-isolating and what to do. This all sounds fairly voluntary, depends upon who has chosen to download the app for their own protection (and those of others, of course), and putatively they have control on the data of movements and contacts being gathered through the app by certain privacy protection mechanisms. To a significant extent, this is a matter of what sort of data is being gathered. The exploitation of data is limited not only by encryption but also by gathering only as much data as is needed to serve the purpose of tracking possible infection contact-points – so even the service providers' ability to exploit this is limited. The app is mandated and distributed through government agencies (it is backed by several governments), who seemingly do not have access to the data on contacts, thus protecting privacy of data. However, several data privacy watchers have expressed concerns about its effect on privacy regulation, as a recent *Wired* article I read detailed. Some governments (such as France) are asking Google and Apple to relax the privacy protection measures so that they can protect their citizens the better.

The Indian government has launched its own Aarogya Setu app, which is announced on its website as follows:

> The Government of India has launched Aarogya Setu, a mobile application aimed to connect health services and we the people of India in our combined fight against COVID-19. The App will augment GoI's initiatives in proactively reaching out to and informing the users about the potential risk of infection, best practices and relevant medical advisories pertaining to the containment of COVID-19 pandemic. The App is privacy-first by design and is currently available in 11 different languages. With Aarogya Setu, let us take a step forward to protecting ourselves, our family & loved ones.[4]

Some might wonder about the contradiction between GoI 'proactively reaching out and informing the users' and the app being 'privacy-first by design'. Obviously, the app is not designed to protect your privacy *from* the GoI; the GoI will protect your privacy while protecting you by design. A Bloomberg Quint article I chanced upon observed, among other things, that this app gathers more data than is needed – than, for instance, the Trace Together app (it seems to be called 'scope creep', which seems to me a nice creepy phrase).[5]

The newspapers today reported on plans being drawn up by the government on standard operational procedures (SOP) after the lockdown is relaxed.[6] One of the key measures proposed is to make the Aarogya Setu app compulsory for all employed in the e-commerce sector (so the bosses in Amazon and Flipkart will have to ensure that all their employees have the app downloaded on their devices). Compulsion would also apply to anyone using public transport which involves security checks (to protect security workers), such as to access the airports or the Delhi Metro. It might well turn out that compulsion attaches to so many categories of citizens that eventually not many are left out. That's what happened by steps with the Aadhaar biometric identity numbers, which began in 2009 as optional and ended up becoming compulsory with the legislation to back compulsion.

Compulsion raises some interesting questions. To begin with, to leave Delhi and get on a flight, I might need to have a smartphone with the app downloaded. Or to go from A to B within Delhi by the metro.

Milena Katsarska (22 April 2020, Plovdiv, Bulgaria)

As far as I have read about those apps, there it is: a way not only to track and manage populations but a way to harden that 1-m bubble territory around a person. It goes both ways in desirably assisting governments to trace contact paths (social–life networks), but it is also marketed as a way to protect yourself and that territory of the 1-m bubble around you. Before long, perhaps alert signals will be going off signalling potential danger in simple proximity; it doesn't matter any longer proximity to whom. Among the other things (data privacy, government monitoring and surveillance, etc.), that is sure to modify and habituate people's behaviour in certain ways.

I think I have mentioned earlier that in the race to be the best and the first (a painstakingly constructed national self-image to be proud of) in the Covid-19 'era', Bulgarian IT developers put forward a local app, Virusafe, as early as April 4.[7] Actually, Bulgarian IT technicians had developed the app earlier. During a Boyko briefing on April 4, it was presented as useful, as a service provided for free by the genius of Bulgarian IT specialists to help the government and citizens. You can download it from the government website designed for Covid-19 matters and news. I should read up on the Indian app to see how it compares. But we are indeed talking of both location and personal information being only accessible to: (1) law enforcement, for usefully tracking quarantine observation – a bit like an ankle monitor for home arrests; (2) the regional health services with direct lines to the emergency HQ for epidemic modelling – detecting clusters that could lead to effective cordons sanitaire; and (3) capabilities of inputting your data (temperature, symptoms, etc.) that are also directly available to your GP so that this primary health contact can undertake care of an increased cohort. I have no idea how many people in Bulgaria have voluntarily downloaded the app thus far or whether it is required for those that test positive. I haven't heard any loud noises in either protest or congratulation from the authorities.

The thing to bear in mind is that most of us are already habituated to using such apps without bothering about it. Whatever business opportunities are there in apps that give you traffic congestion information or dating opportunities, they involve people giving information on their relative locations.

My guess is that one will have in-app purchases of levels (up to premium or super star) giving access to a variety of 'services' additional to risky contact tracking. It might offer real-time calculation of safest, contagion-free routes or spots, for instance. It could become an event planner's 'must have' assistant for planning weddings, conferences, concerts, and what not. Besides government coercion, work-environment coercion may play its part but also voluntary participation in 'the club' of the initiated. Contact information and a health profile with location are yet another tool for strategic and targeted advertising and publicity campaigns – commercial and political.

Virusafe is placed on the Unified Portal for the Bulgarian Covid-19 Situation that bears the hallmarks of the state (coat of arms).[8] It is within the domain of the Ministry of Health and presented as a separate space of the 'operation HQ'. It is available to download from Google Play and the Apple Store. The announcement on that portal states the following in bold: 'The aim of this app is to provide an opportunity to all residing in the Republic of Bulgaria to participate and assist by inputting their data and stating their condition daily'.

Peter H. Tu (23 April 2020, Niskayuna, New York State, United States)

I started keeping track of days using the time-honored tradition of scratching a line for every day and then crossing the lines on the fifth day. However, like my trip to Alcatraz, the prisonlike novelty wears off – so the days are starting to blend.

At this moment, upper management has tasked me with putting together some sort of app-driven device that can be used to assure other passengers of a plane that you are not in a position to infect them. Options include: a note from your primary care physician, some sort of contact-tracing application, the ability to detect symptoms, and the use of physiological and avatar-driven interactions to come up with a machine-learning-based classifier.

I was listening to how contact tracing is done in South Korea. During the MERS epidemic, the government refused to divulge which hospitals were taking care of MERS patients. The population was upset and in a vigilante kind of way figured it out for itself and simply posted this information. So the government did a 180 and revealed everything. This is now the strategy for contact tracing. While they do not publish the names of infected people, they do publish their 2–3 week history so that people will read it, digest it, and come forward. The argument is that the published narrative has to be compelling enough to jog people's memories. But there are repercussions. One example is the following: a 20-year-old female working as a bartender at Jack's Bar and Grill has been infected. The following is a list of her activities. Some of these items may be a restaurant, others might involve an overnight liaison. . . . Of course it does not take long for social media to ferret out who the individual is, and before long various forms of shaming naturally ensue.

Not sure where this will all go.

Richard Allen (25 April 2020, Birmingham, United Kingdom)

The virus has made its mark in our little street. The man next door has been ill in the last week – ill enough to have the paramedics in the night – but has stayed at home and we think is now recovering. He's quite young but also a consultant at one of the local hospitals, so presumably picked it up there. Next door but one has been more serious and sad. The couple there are our age and both pretty active, but M★ has quite well-advanced Parkinson's disease. His partner M is a leading light in the Bach Choir and picked up the bug, along with 18 others, at a gathering just before the lockdown. She passed it to M★, and it seemed they were getting through it, but M★ was more seriously affected and has died. They were also active in the local church, so apart from not being able to be very sociable with M, the street has not been able to show our affection for M★ in a funeral. I guess there'll be a memorial after things have 'unlocked'. I think it's been very confusing for M because she had made the decision to care for M★ at home in the future and they are partway through having the house adapted. So, on the one hand, that's not happening, but, on the other hand, there is a measure of relief that M★ will be spared the more advanced stages of Parkinson's.

And generally, how depressed one feels about the inadequacies of the government in preparing for and managing the crisis, and how embarrassed by the sight of Dominic Raab standing in front of the flags – definitely the last resort of the scoundrel. And how further depressing as the curtain of coronavirus is drawn aside a little to reveal the whole Brexit disaster still lurking there. It's perfectly extraordinary that Johnson's absence is so accepted; he surely has been absent from office for much longer than he has been present now. And how irritating to see the 'scientists' casting a cloak over the government's inadequacies. They seem cut from the same cloth as the people running the NHS, who cheerfully designed a plan for fewer beds as a cover for the government's cost cutting, without any real attempt at forward vision.

I won't rant further. Practically we are coping. We have worries about shopping but are doing OK and have had two deliveries from Sainsbury's. We bake our own bread with a bread maker and were troubled by the lack of flour but have managed to get a big bag online. Our main lack comes from the absence of the farmers' markets, where we get real cheese and real sausages. We haven't quite worked out how to manage that but are tempted by (pricey!) online offerings. I've worked my way through the Ferrante Neapolitan quartet of novels and am wondering what to read next. We had our book group yesterday by Zoom and read *The Watchmaker of Filigree Street*. I recommend it as a jolly but also intelligent and imaginative read. It's our turn to choose the book for next time, so – after discussion – we have chosen *The Plague*, which is curiously out of stock! We learn that Penguin UK have reprinted their edition seven times during the pandemic; were they not confident the pandemic would last?

Ayan-Yue Gupta (25 April 2020, London, United Kingdom)

Having nightmarish visions of this going on forever.

Do you remember nudge psychology? Seems the compulsion vs voluntary use of these apps mirrors the difference between directly authoritarian governing and one-dimensional-man-style authoritarianism filtered through a proxy of hollow voluntarism. Maybe the slide towards more total forms of control is inevitable, and the path back to pre-Covid levels of self-possession has gone. There will only be more pandemics in the future, and maybe the only way to deal with them, aside from a complete shift away from hollowing out public healthcare, is through more totalizing forms of control.

Notes

1 Edward T. Hall, *The Hidden Dimension* (New York: Doubleday, 1966).
2 Henri Lefebvre, *The Production of Space*, trans. Donald Nicholson-Smith (Oxford: Blackwell, 1991 [1974]).
3 Agnieszka Sorokowska, Piotr Sorokowski, Peter Hilpert, Katarzyna Cantarero, Thomas Frackowiak, Khodabakhsh Ahmadi, Ahmad M. Alghraibeh, Ricd Aryeetey, Anna Bertoni, Karim Bettache, et al., 'Preferred interpersonal distances: A global comparison', *Journal of Cross-Cultural Psychology* 48: 4, 2017, 577–92, DOI: 10.1177/0022022117698039.
4 'Aarogya Setu app: COVID-19 tracker launched to alert you and keep you safe. Download now!' www.mygov.in/task/aarogya-setu-app-covid-19-tracker-launched-alert-you-and-keep-you-safe-download-now/ (accessed 1 June 2020).
5 Anand Venkatanarayan, 'Covid-19: How the Aarogya Setu app handles your data', *Bloomberg Quint*, 17 April 2020, www.bloombergquint.com/coronavirus-outbreak/covid-19-how-the-aarogya-setu-app-handles-your-data (accessed 1 June 2020).
6 'From staffing to transport, govt details SOP for firms', *Times of India*, 16 April 2020, https://timesofindia.indiatimes.com/business/india-business/from-staffing-to-transport-govt-details-sop-for-firms/articleshow/75171682.cms (accessed 1 June 2020).
7 'Scalefocus team joins forces to help in the fight against COVID-19', *Scalefocus*, 4 April 2020, www.scalefocus.com/news/scalefocus-team-joins-forces-to-help-in-the-fight-against-covid-19 (accessed 2 June 2020).
8 https://coronavirus.bg/bg/ (accessed 2 June 2020).

10

TAX THE RICH

Summary: *An unofficial report from the heart of the Indian government's financial offices caused a brief stir in the media. It recommended a range of strategies for financing the government's response to the Covid-19 crisis, from increased taxation of the super-rich to supporting migrant workers and boosting the public healthcare system. The government was quick to disown it. The measures proposed and the government's response are discussed in some of the interventions here. That leads into broader observations on the current socioeconomic order and on the authors' sense of this in early May as the Covid-19 crisis continued.*

Suman Gupta (27 April 2020, Delhi, India)

A news report

My waning interest in the newspapers found unexpected stimulation this morning from an unusual news item. It was reported that some officers of the Indian Revenue Service (IRS) had released a report which ruffled the feathers of their ministerial and bureaucratic bosses. The IRS is a central government body dealing with both direct and indirect taxation policy under the Ministry of Finance, answering to the statutory bodies the Central Board of Direct Taxes (CBDT) and the Central Board of Indirect Taxes and Customs (CBIC). The newspaper at hand that I read, *Hindustan Times*,[1] reported that a group of IRS officers had released an 'ill-conceived report' through the IRS Association which 'suggested raising income-tax rate up to 40%, imposing a super-rich tax and levy a 4% Covid-19 relief cess to rebuild the economy post-coronavirus pandemic'. The government had 'summarily' rejected this 'ill-conceived report'. Two finance ministry officials, who requested that they not be named, described the report as an 'irresponsible act' which might have had deleterious effects on the economy and caused panic in the market; luckily the market was closed when it appeared. They announced that a departmental enquiry would be conducted against the persons responsible.

That such a report could emerge from the heart of the GoI's Ministry of Finance is as extraordinary as this obviously nervous ministry response (even the officials laying out the ministry's severe condemnation 'requested anonymity'!). Naturally, I took to the web; the news item has appeared in much the same terms in most national dailies and international business columns. In fact, on Twitter, the IRS Association had already issued a disclaimer, pretty much when the news report was filed: 'The paper FORCE by 50 young IRS officers suggesting policy measures had been forwarded by IRSA to CBDT for consideration. It does not purport to represent the official views of the entire IRS, or the IT department'.[2] Twitter feeds were buzzing with the story in financial and business and political circles, most recommending that the heads of the offending IRS officers should roll. The next step was to look for a full text of the report, which wasn't difficult to find.

The Indian Revenue Service association report

The report,[3] published under the IRS, GoI insignia, is written by 50 IRS officers of the batches who joined between 2014 and 2019. They describe their initiative thus:

> As the nation went into a strategic and defensive huddle, 50 plus young officers of Indian Revenue Service (IT) came together to leverage their combined knowledge, expertise and love for India and find some more solutions, suggestions and options that will help with the treatment for the economic pain that the country is suffering. Focusing thoughts and efforts on their domain knowledge and expertise, this volunteering initiative tried to identify actionable areas to mobilise revenue while protecting taxpayers' welfare as a fiscal policy response in general and response of direct taxes administration in particular.

The report then does several things: (1) gives the background on GoI's response to the Covid crisis thus far in fiscal terms and some comparative information on responses in other countries; (2) outlines measures for increasing tax income under current circumstances so that GoI's response can be more robust; (3) outlines measures for compensating poor and marginal workers, giving tax breaks to MSMEs, shoring up the public health service against the increased funding raised through (2); and (4) enumerates measures for regulating and policing the proposed taxation regime.

The news universally focused on (2), the measures recommended for raising funding through taxation, and gave short shrift to (3), compensatory measures. No doubt (2) was the bit that made the Ministry so nervous. However, as the report argued, raising funding through taxation (2) is a necessary counterpart to compensatory measures (3). The news media largely stuck to highlighting (2) as the more sensational and panic-inducing aspect of the report (for GoI anyway) and parroted the Ministry's floundering and scared condemnation. Arguably the Ministry protested too much and actually aroused interest in the report. Let me focus on (2) also, since that's what the GoI is nervous about.

Recommendations

Here are the key points made about how GoI should raise money for the Covid crisis through taxation – some direct quotations from the report follow:

1. In times like these, the so called 'super rich' have a higher obligation towards ensuring the larger public good. This is for multiple reasons – they enjoy a higher capacity to pay with significantly higher levels of disposable incomes compared with the rest, they have a higher stake in ensuring the economy springs back into action, and their current levels of wealth itself is a product of the social contract between the state and its citizens. Most high-income earners still have the luxury of working from home, and the wealthy can fall back upon their wealth to cope with the temporary shock. . . . Therefore, this segment of the population can be taxed through two alternative means, both of which can be imposed for a limited, fixed period of time: * *raising highest slab rate to 40% for total income levels above a min. threshold of Rs. 1 cr/ Or/* * re-introduction of the wealth tax for those with net wealth of Rs. 5 crores or more.*

2. Increase the surcharge applicable to the Higher income Foreign Companies having a Branch Office/ Permanent Establishment in India. The said surcharge has not been revised for some time now, and with companies operating in India and deriving profits through their PEs, it is time that a flourishing market like India with its huge prospects flexes its customer-base muscle.

3. As per the current law, specified class of companies are required to spend 2 per cent of their average net profits as CSR [Corporate Social Responsibility, usually with tax breaks], failing which the Board has to incorporate the reasons for such failure in its report. A scheme can be proposed to provide a one-time opportunity to the companies to contribute a portion of their unspent CSR funds until FY 2019–20 to PM CARES Fund and utilize a portion of such unspent money for their business purpose. . . . Contributions to PM CARES Fund and CM Relief Funds should be allowed to be counted as CSR not only for the current FY but also for FY 2021–22.

4. A tax on MNEs [Multinational Enterprises] on the lines of Base erosion anti-abuse tax (BEAT) of US can be introduced. It will

impose an additional tax liability on certain corporations that make base-eroding payments (e.g., interest, royalty, etc.) to foreign related parties.

5. Inheritance tax is levied mostly in developed countries, at rates as high as 55%. In India, it was in force till 1985, payable on a slab basis. Inheritance tax, if reintroduced, is expected to reduce concentration of wealth, widen the tax base and enhance revenue, and play its part in bridging the wealth inequality divide. More importantly, such a tax may eventually lead to reduction in tax rates.

6. In the issue of capital gains and in the case of OCI [Overseas Citizens of India], the capital gains accruing out of the inherited properties of the oversees citizens to be raised by 10% margin from the current rate. The reason being that on various stages in the life of the OCI, the inherited properties and the persons holding them would have benefitted from the facilities and subsidies offered by the Government of India.

7. The consumption of online services, especially web streaming services such as Netflix, Amazon Prime, Zoom, etc. and the increased dependence on online commerce has made this sector flourish. The increased business of these e commerce/ online streaming/ web services companies provides an opportunity to increase the said tax [Equalization Tax] rates by 1%, i.e. from 6% to 7% for ad services, and from 2% to 3% for e-commerce.

8. Just like it was done in the case of LPG subsidy where many well off people voluntarily surrendered their LPG [liquefied petroleum gas] subsidy benefits [i.e. to buy the product at market rather than government subsidized prices], the tax department can encourage the superrich and those willing, to give up at least one tax subsidy/ tax deduction/ tax concession for only a year – for e.g. an individual could voluntarily opt for giving up his/her 80C deduction for a year.

These are the measures suggested for raising tax revenue to deal with the Covid-19 crisis. The following section of the report on how this funding should be used is of equal if not more interest, but I don't go into this now. Apparently these increased taxation measures are the ones that made GoI nervous. But, who knows, perhaps it is actually the prospect of improving the lot of the poor and the marginalized, shoring up the public health service, giving lifelines to MSMEs that makes GoI nervous. The optimistic view taken in the report is:[4]

The Covid stimulus package announced by the Government of India thus far amounts to 0.8% of GDP. *Prima facie*, this pales in comparison with 11% in the case of US, 15% in the case of UK, and 16% in the case of Malaysia. However, India's Covid stimulus package was not the end, it was just the beginning. If additional revenues can be mobilized through some of the steps proposed above, the Government will have the legroom to significantly expand the scope and size of the stimulus/relief package without making a huge dent on its fiscal deficit position.

Nuances

So, here are two questions: What is it about these measures that causes such concern up there? And how might this story unfold, whether or not it stays news? Some nuances to this story suggest themselves to me.

1   Obviously, the report recommends redistribution conducted by the state, GoI, to deal with the Covid crisis. Judging from news reports, the immediate response of the Ministry was that taxing rich individuals and businesses would make the elites unhappy, they might reduce their investments and business activities – less FDI, less 'Made in India', fewer lucrative public/private and private/private partnerships, drops in share value of Indian-owned businesses in international exchanges, downgrading of 'ease of business' . . . less of all the things that the current BJP GoI and its sponsors have been working for so energetically. It is in the nature of neoliberal arrangements that states and corporations/elites have a symbiotic relationship of mutual dependency to serve their mutual interests – of concentration of power and money. However, in this symbiotic relationship, the corporations/elites have the upper hand, since they can shift operations to another geopolitical territory, but the state can't really move the geopolitical territory that has appointed it. So, in an immediate way, the nervousness of GoI is due to fear of the corporations/elites, the dominant brokers of neoliberalism.

2   Perhaps as importantly, it is fear of the Other of neoliberalism. But what is the Other? In fact, there are several versions of the Other. One that is raised by this document immediately is a kind of centre (progressive/neo-Keynesian) liberal formation which focuses on inequality and adjustments in tax regimes alongside increased public investments/projects to equalize. It brings to mind quite vividly the Occupy Movement of, mainly, 2011–2012, and its slogan, 'The 1% and the 99%'. Behind that focus on inequality lay the work of some economists, which was later marked by the remarkable market and media success of books like Thomas Piketty's *Capital in the Twenty-First Century* (2014 [2013]), in the popular appeal of Joseph Stiglitz's *The Price of Inequality* (2012) and Paul Krugman's *End This Depression Now!* (2012), and in Anthony B. Atkinson's *Inequality: What Can Be Done?* (2015).[5] Before the Occupy Movement, a series of papers from around 2000 by Emmanuel Saez, Thomas Piketty, Facundo Alvaredo, Anthony Atkinson, Michael Veall, Gabriel Zucman, and others provided the line that converged into that movement (and the rising popularity of Bernie Sanders in the United States). These young IRS officers sound as if they might be straightforwardly aligned in their thinking to Occupy Movement ideologues, though in fact they are quite modest in their recommendations.

For instance, the recommendation to raise upper-level income tax to 40% for three years shouldn't make anyone blink (in the United Kingdom, it is set at 40% upper level and 45% at the highest level; in France, it is correspondingly 41% and 45%; in Germany, it is 42% for the highest, etc.) – Saez, Piketty, and Atkinson would recommend the highest levels at 60% and above indefinitely. Nor is a blanket increase on high-level capital gains, which particularly pay the rich, recommended (currently set at a very modest 10%–15% in India, dependent on whether the investment is long or short term).

3   A fallout of the redistributive thinking is that it effectively increases the footprint of the public sector in the economy, though that is not really stressed in the report. In fact, every measure is phrased tentatively enough not to emphasize that. Therein lurks the spectre of socialism, the natural enemy of the religious nationalist formation that is the GoI now. The recommendation to reintroduce inheritance tax, to shore up the public health service at the expense of the vast private health service (the custom of the affluent and middle classes is exclusively focused there) is apt to seem to this GoI as a slippery slope of renationalizing sectors or returning to a sort-of-socialist Planning Commission stage of the Indian economy. This spectre gives a hint of what might happen to this courageous group of 50 young IRS officers, beyond a departmental investigation into the propriety of publicly releasing this document. On the Hindu right, they would now seem to fit the conspiracy model of 'urban naxals' perfectly, as laid out at length, for instance, in Vivek Agnihotri's film *Buddha in a Traffic Jam* (2014) and then his book *Urban Naxals* (2018)[6] – which construct an anti-national communist enemy within, which has infiltrated academia, media, and high government offices. It is unlikely that the fact that this group of IRS officers have not tried to be surreptitious, quite the contrary, will give them any advantage. A whole legal process of persecuting alleged 'urban naxals' has emerged since 2014, which can lock up (even amidst lockdown) almost any progressive person who doesn't buy into uncritical religious nationalism. This group may well find itself pegged as such.

4   Fear of the people: the poor, the marginalized, the migrant day-wage worker, the small trader and petty shop-floor worker, the cart vendors, the crafts persons, and so on – all on edge as their livelihoods and meagre savings vanish under the Covid-19 lockdowns.

Peter H. Tu (28 April 2020, Niskayuna, New York State, United States)

The IRS 50 have certainly touched a nerve. Your nuance section hits the general reactions one gets whenever one suggests that the top 1% relinquish some of their treasure: (1) If you tax the rich, they will take their business elsewhere. At the heart of neoliberalism is the desire to make the state sufficiently attractive for the rich. (2) This is a plot put together by the new-left. If given half a chance, the AOCs, the

Bernies, and the Corbyns will take over and run this country into the ground. (3) The slippery slope to socialism – just look at Cuba and Venezuela.

Earlier in the year, a wealth tax was championed by Bernie Sanders and more seriously by Elizabeth Warren. This was mostly to address the question of health-care for all, global warming, and free college. The consultants that were helping Warren with her wealth tax facts and figures made a compelling case. But, as you might imagine, there was a well-orchestrated push-back by the establishment – much like your 1, 2, 3 arguments. I listened to a podcast by one of Warren's wealth tax consultants, who did a pretty good job of refuting most of these arguments. At the end of the day, it comes down to the fact that Warren Buffett pays himself a taxable salary of $100,000, has a net worth of around $70 billion, and pays a lower tax rate than his secretary on his actual wealth growth.[7] Of course, the wealth is just about untaxable.

At this point in time, the Republicans are certainly not suggesting a tax hike on the rich. Their crowning achievement to date was a huge tax cut that resulted in the largest debt ever. Just about all of it went to a reduction in corporate taxes, resulting in stock buybacks and CEO bonuses. As is always the case, just about nothing trickled down. So the answer right now is to print more money. This, of course, devalues assets held with US currency and increases the national debt. The fear of a blossoming debt is that at some point in time, servicing that debt will become so onerous that an administration will seek hyper-inflation as means of debt relief. This hurts anyone who hopes to retire based on savings and/or pensions.

My understanding is that President Nixon arranged for Saudi Arabia to agree to only sell oil for US dollars. In return, US military bases ensure the sovereignty of their regime. This is one of the reasons that American dollars are the currency of choice. If, however, it is continually devalued based on 'just printing', then this opens the door for a new currency of choice to emerge. I have heard speculation that China is attempting to purchase enough gold that would allow it to tie its currency to some sort of gold standard. If successful, such stability might make the RMB very attractive. Of course, international monetary policy is something that I know little to nothing about.

Richard Allen (28 April 2020, Birmingham, United Kingdom)

On the face of it, it's good that a group such as the IRS one still thinks it can put out such a report, although alongside the redistributive aspect there is also a 'tight money' aspect that is perhaps less congenial. I guess you weren't surprised that the Indian government slapped them down, since that's of a piece with most other countries following the US example of borrowing with abandon and ignoring the deficit. That certainly seems the policy in the United Kingdom, where the government is waving money around as though it did grow on the proverbial tree in contrast to previous policies of austerity. There's no doubt a Brexit angle to this. Britain being great again will lead to the pound becoming again the reserve currency of choice as opposed to being a basket case required to pay higher and higher rates on government bonds.

Going back to India and the IRS report, the government's reaction speaks of perhaps: (1) on the one hand, a certain two-facedness whereby the Covid-19 crisis is so significant that the lockdown is justified, while, on the other, carrying on as if it is not important enough to disturb BJP's plans (with their inbuilt fostering of inequality) or (2) a willingness to use the virus outbreak as a cover for the locking out of protests arising from the Citizenship Act and other Hindutva actions. And, of course, there's always the likelihood that the Modi government – like most governments – lives so much in its own rhetoric about the success of its policies that it can't think outside the rhetoric. As we witness in the United Kingdom, where it is sufficient to say that 'our aim' is to ensure there is enough protective clothing for medical workers for that problem to be solved. The prize for that kind of thing, incidentally, goes to Iain Duncan Smith, who wrote recently on Conservative Home, 'Here's to a quiet success in the struggle against the virus – the resilience and robustness of Universal Credit'.[8]

Looking, as I do, at the John Hopkins website,[9] the Coronavirus statistics present India as a bit of a puzzle.

UK: Confirmed cases 154,000; Deaths 20,700; Case Fatality 13.5%; Deaths per 100k population 31.27% (close to the highest)
India: Confirmed cases 27,800; Deaths 881; Case-fatality 3.2%; Deaths per 100k population 0.07%

Given the population size and the size of the country, one might wonder how effectively the Indian government can reliably know these kinds of statistics, though the heritage of the bean-counting Empire might help. That said, and going back to the original point you made, at the moment, Covid-19 is a pretty minor condition. But responding to Covid-19 has the 'advantage' of an international way of responding and an international discourse that is simple. Somehow we can beat this virus by a lockdown where we can't lock down mosquitoes or the causes of respiratory diseases or malnutrition. Does the Modi government offer any nuanced commentary on its position?

Sebastian Schuller (30 April 2020, Munich, Germany)

Let me organize my thoughts by thinking through an example that I consider of paramount importance in this context of disaster – triage.

Wikipedia tells me that triage,[10] though practiced for thousands of years, was formalized and regulated during World War I, when medical personnel had to decide which of the injured to treat and which to leave to their fate. Here, then, we find a practice – not to help people in need – that is considered scandalous, even outlawed under the normality of liberal democratic society, but which is allowed and considered necessary under the state of exception of war. But this licence to transgress depends on two conditions: (1) there must be declared a state of exception; that is, the rules of liberal society are suspended for a period of time; and (2) those who enact triage are licensed to do so – they are military personnel, representatives of the state. Otherwise, even in exceptional circumstances, we tend to be scandalized by the abandonment of the needy. Consider mountaineers who are forced to leave an injured comrade behind: even if their action is not tantamount to a crime, it is likely to be seen as presenting an ethical problem. Mountaineers are not representatives of state, and an expedition is a private matter. In any case, triage in the 20th century is a biopolitical practice that is nonetheless of public interest. After World War I, for instance, we see accounts, literary and non-literary, that mourn the brutality of the war and denounce triage as a failure of the state.

Triage under Covid-19: currently, we find ourselves in a global state of exception, and we do not know when or whether this will end. And we find ourselves confronted with a similar problem that the medics of World War I had to face: the capacity to treat the sick does not suffice; triage is needed.

There is, however, a significant difference from triage in World War I here. This state of exception is no longer limited to the rims of society; it is comprehensive and global. We no longer have normal zones as a contrast for the exceptionality that legitimizes triage. At present, the normality is the exception and vice versa. But, in addition to that, there is a second difference. Those who practice triage no longer necessarily or clearly represent the state. They are not military personnel, they are medical workers – often of private institutions. The state may licence them to enact control over life, to practice triage (which, for example, is what this law in the United Kingdom that allows doctors to issue DNR forms at will is about) and grant them immunity. But that does not alter the fact that private organizations have replaced or been co-opted by state bodies – a matter I return to shortly.

This rationale is not specific to Covid-19, though it appears to be accepted more widely and worked with more speedily now. However, we have seen this tendency appearing variously for some time. Three examples come to mind. (1) Security companies, a.k.a. mercenaries, have been fulfilling the military obligations of states since the early 1990s, whether that's in the United States hiring Blackwater (or whatever the company is called now) to fight in Iraq or whether, as in Germany, barracks are guarded by private security firms or German cities hire private companies to patrol the streets at night because of shortages in the police force. (2) In the case of climate change, various inter- and binational treaties since the early 1990s agree that this problem has to be addressed at a global scale. But the measures taken consist more or less in founding a niche market for emissions: companies can trade emission certificates; some even plant trees in rainforests in order to create emission certificates. Thus, a problem of governmental regulation is 'outsourced' to the private sector and its agents. (3) With regard to law-making: in Germany, for example, it is now a common practice for federal as well as regional ministries to engage private law firms to actually write the text of the law. These firms are sometimes connected to lobby groups or even individual companies but nevertheless do the job of secretaries of state.

We might assume that this is tantamount to the logic of neoliberalism: everything should be marketized. And no doubt, this tendency itself is due to the neoliberal logic and agenda, so widely discussed since Foucault's late 1970s lectures in *The Birth of Biopolitics*.[11] And yet, I feel that on the whole these processes and tendencies tend towards something other than the current neoliberal order.

Actually, what I presented as the replacement of the state through the private sphere is an imprecise description of what is actually taking place. On the one side, of course, we see these tendencies. What was the obligation of the public sphere becomes a function of the private sector. On the other side, the private sector tends also to become the obligation of the public. Bailout programs, for example, are a way through which the state mingles with the market. In the healthcare sector, we see – of course with national variations – how the state, legal bodies, insurance companies, healthcare providers, and so on are mingled together and become impossible to extricate at times. We may say: the public becomes privatized *as the public*. The state does not disappear, as the fantasies of libertarianism would have it, but it becomes at one with capital; the private and the public sphere are merging.

This is the case with triage in times of Covid-19. The triaging agents are private agents, but as private agents they fulfil the duty of the state and are licensed to do so. A healthcare provider can decide over life and death according to a very simple rationale: are there enough beds? In other words, the biopolitical power of the state is still there, but it is now no longer a political decision – to my knowledge, no parliament decided openly to let the 'weak' die – but a simple question of supply and demand. A question of the public and yet not-public logic of the market.

The shortage of beds, equipment, medicines, tests, and so on – the inability to effectively act in the Covid-19 crisis – are of course consequences of the privatizing of healthcare in the first place, as we know. But this is not a question to be raised in a significant way at the moment. If I say, as a militant activist, 'The privatization of healthcare made triage necessary' – I would nevertheless fail to address the reality of triage. I address its structural reasons, but in doing so I merely encounter its reality. It is impossible to demand an end to triage as the logic of triage is not due to public considerations but is now the inevitable consequence of the marketized logic of healthcare capitalism.

This may be one of the reasons for the apolitical effects of Covid-19, which was discussed in an earlier intervention. The making public of the private and the privatization of the public result in situations where politics can disappear. It is, as I said, at the moment impossible to criticize triage as it is practiced, as there are no alternatives to it; we have to accept its current reality. Yet, if we do so, we accept the reality of a structural presence of the market rationale. No singular, conscientious political decision made triage necessary, but its necessity flows out of the unpersonal and (seemingly) apolitical rationality of the system; it is a structural consequence of our reality. We have of course the option of *deferring* it, by social distancing, by putting in more beds in hospitals, and so on. But we can't address it as a matter of political decisions. The situation that led to the implementation of triage is due to a complex set of decisions and ideologies that led to the absolutism of the market in the public sphere.

The rule of experts, for example, can be seen in this light. In the case of Covid-19, virology replaces the political public, simply because there is nothing to be done about the political misery at the moment; there is no way out of triage. These phenomena, even if deplorable, are consequences of a reality beyond the political: they are apolitical in nature – that is, insofar as these measures are not subject to an expressed political will. Instead, they appear as results and structural moments of the privatization of the public, of the induction of a market rationale into the political sphere and the subsequent integration of state and capital. Just as an enterprise may only act according to the market, to act within this framework means to follow these structures and their interpretations through a horde of experts.

And this is what happens now: in all fields, people are discussing Covid-19 – educational, economic and healthcare politics. But the way in which it is discussed is radically apolitical. Take Trump: if he calls for a 'liberation' of states under lockdown, he does not present us with a coherent political programme (such as Social Darwinism), he refers to business expertise that shows how necessary it is to end the lockdown. In other words, his political decision is not political in the strong sense of the word. It is not bound to an ideology, to an idea of any sort; rather, the political moment rests in the evaluation of competing expertises. Just as a captain of industry may choose between different analyses and assessments of the market, Trump and indeed all political leaders everywhere do the same. They accept the structural reality of something beyond their control and act only within the confines of different analyses of these structures. This is true for political debate *in toto*. The structure itself is not an object of debate.

With these observations in mind, let me consider the situation of the Government of India and the young IRS officers who wrote the offending report.

It seems clear to me that neither the GoI nor these IRS officers address the structural reality of public capital as such. Their difference is little more than a contradiction within the current system. That is, both accept the structures of an omnipresent market rationale but understand that the current situation is a global disaster.

The GoI now seems basically to act in the traditional neoliberal way. The disaster is something – and I emphasize this point – that is outside the control of market forces, so it is necessary to let it happen, no matter what, as it cannot be addressed by the structures of the market. So, the only actions to be taken are those that preserve the status quo.

The young IRS officers, however, understand that the disaster is something that endangers the existing order. So what they propose is a radicalization of the current tendency of aligning the public sphere with capital. Their proposals basically call for a higher rate of public spending – that is, for an acceleration of the integration of state and capital. As I said, the market should be replaced by the state. The consequence of this is that the elites are reduced to rentiers of the structures of a public sphere capitalism that profit from the system while the system carries on, following its immanent drive.

So, we have two alternatives, and this appears on a global scale: either there is disaster neoliberalism, where the failure of the system will be met by authoritarian measures, or, as I dub it, post-liberalism, where the public sphere finally is identical with the market. Yet both alternatives share the same apolitical worldview. They are just variants on how to adapt society to the structures of a universal market that cannot be grasped within political discourse any longer. What made the liberal state liberal – the regulation of the market forces – has been perverted and inverted in both alternatives. The market forces regulate the state. The right-wing neoliberal leaves things as they are, while the progressive, post-liberal alternative seeks to overcome this by merging the state and the market.

So, the question seems to be: how to find a language that is able to address the structure of global capitalism and to challenge it? It seems to me that it is necessary to re-invent politics – in the sense that we must find ways to think about, address, and attack these situations, like triage, in a way that lays bare their political meaning, their inner constitution as outflows of the universalization of the market.

Suman Gupta (3 May 2020, Delhi, India)

Here's how things are looking around me now, where I live.

My evening walk takes me past the dense spontaneous agglomeration of a bazaar, Madhu Vihar, with tiny tiny shops packed tightly together along a warren of narrow lanes, which are usually packed with bodies rippling up and down. Nowadays it is deserted, desultory and forlorn, with a waiting air in there. Some of the narrow lanes have barricades in front of them. Along these lanes, the hungry wait in orderly queues on both sides, carefully spaced 1 metre from each other, squatting or kneeling all the way up. Some have face masks; most just cover their faces with a hanky or a corner of the sari. Up there somewhere, there is a charitable religious foundation; the waiting hungry are being subjected to pious bhajans on a crackling loudspeaker. I suppose if the waiting hungry can put up with it long enough, they will get food. They don't talk much to each other.

Along the 2 or 3 km of my unlovely evening walk, I cross women in twos or threes squatting on the pavements or just standing at the end of roads, not doing much. They call out to me asking for some help, begging. Some hold babies. Some are very young, teenagers, some elderly. I guess these are the domestic workers not getting paid, or maybe the wives of daily wage earners who aren't getting wages. Begging is one way to try to get along.

The Delhi Chief Minister Arvind Kejriwal appeared on TV this evening.[12] The central government yesterday announced some relaxation across the country, according to whether they are designated as red, orange, or green zones – and extended the lockdown to 16 May. Delhi is all red. Kejriwal said all the relaxations possible for a red zone would be allowed in Delhi during this phase of the lockdown. All government offices will open and a significant number of businesses, possibly non-essential movement will be allowed between 7am and 7pm, but all malls, restaurants, parks, and so on will remain closed, and buses, trains, planes, taxis, and so on will continue not to operate. Household servants can go back to work. Some alcohol shops will open. And so on. He said that it's not so much that the contagion is diminishing. The total lockdown has been useful in slowing its spread. And it has given the state government time to prepare. There are now adequate supplies to deal with cases to come. More hospital beds have been set up. There are 97 containment zones which will remain sealed, and no relaxation will happen there. Ever more testing will continue, and the latest thing, plasma injections. But the fact is that we can't really sit back and expect the contagion to simply go away, for cases to drop to zero. Meanwhile, many people are starving despite the government setting up food programmes for the poor. The government is itself running out of money. In April, the Delhi government got nothing and spent much. If this continues, there will be no government. So, we'll just have to learn to live with this virus. We will keep social distancing and try hard to not do the things that are dangerous, but we have to gradually get back to work. Otherwise we can't carry on. In fact, he is appealing to the central government to consider Delhi a green area except for the 97 sealed containment zones so that Delhi can get back to life. This relaxation will mean more cases. We have to be ready for that. We have prepared for that. That's what the lockdown has enabled . . .

Fabio Akcelrud Durão (6 May 2020, São Carlos, São Paulo State, Brazil)

With Covid-19, the situation in Brazil, which was already delicate enough, acquired an extreme degree of complexity and urgency. It is useful, for the sake of clarity, to think of three distinct but interrelated crises.

The first crisis is that of the virus itself, of course, which appears in much the same way all over the world. Brazil had time to get prepared but failed to do so properly. Measures were taken on an ad hoc basis, always at the last minute. The incompetence of the public health setup derives from a neoliberal mindset that can't conceive of the government taking a decisive leading role. One begins to glimpse the dramatic character of the Brazilian predicament when one realizes that sheer incompetence must be differentiated from the boycott of treatment and palliative measures.

The second crisis is a political one. The president has been doing everything he can to stage a coup and close Congress and the Supreme Court in the middle of the pandemic. There are two factors encouraging Bolsonaro to precipitate this crisis. On the one hand, he believes that the recession and probable depression to come will annul his chances of being re-elected. So, he is pitting everything he has against social distancing and in favour of business as usual. That way, when the disease is over and the economic situation is dire, he can claim that he is not responsible. On the other hand, investigations are under way that may implicate him and his sons in several crimes,[13] not only of corruption but also linked to the assassination in March 2018 of Marielle Franco (the feminist activist who was city councillor in Rio for PSOL).[14] These explain the timing: Bolsonaro is pushing for chaos so that he can appear as the voice of order and stop investigations into his family. Whether he has the muscle to really bring about the coup is an open question. Though support from the military is uncertain, Bolsonaro does have the support of the lower strata of state police and armed forces (which would have to rebel against their superiors to advance with him), factions of organized criminal organizations (known in Brazil as militias), and a big chunk of Evangelicals. It is not easy to listen to a Congressman threatening civil war if Bolsonaro is ousted, even if it was a bluff, as Roberto Jefferson was recorded and reported doing on 29 April.[15]

The third crisis is economic. The result of the two previous crises is going to be an unheard-of degree of immiseration in the country. Congress forced the federal government to offer a monthly support of 600 reais (a little more than 100 US dollars) to the poor. This measure is also being implemented imperfectly – partly from incompetence and partly due to ill will – and it is doubtful how much of the resources are reaching the poor people. During the 19th century, epidemics were much easier to deal with: the rich secluded themselves in their fortified spaces and waited for the poor to assimilate the disease and die, and then returned to their normal lives. This would be Bolsonaro's dream. If there is a stock market for the lives of the poor, their bonds have never been so low.

So, to sum up, now we have states and municipalities having to struggle on their own against the virus *and* the federal government. The rich are in their houses waiting for the pandemic to pass, while the poor are forced to work and hope they will not die of Covid-19 today or of hunger tomorrow. An armed insurrection against democracy would only add a third kind of death in this necropolis Brazil has become.

John Seed (6 May 2020, London, United Kingdom)

A beautiful summer afternoon a day or two ago, walking along a tree-lined path across Cannon Hill Common: a young woman and her two kids – boy and girl, maybe eight and ten years old – coming towards me. About 10 yards ahead she shouted at them and pulled them off the path, hugged them to her and glared at me as I walked past. It was a glare. There was nowhere else for me to go, and the path was public and wide enough for us to pass comfortably. The irony was, of course, that of the four people present, I was the most vulnerable and her precious kids the least. Welcome to the new normal.

I wonder if she was reflecting on the sacrifices she thought she was making too? In the counting-houses of the spirit, the imaginary debts incurred during the lockdown are already being calculated. I wonder what interest will be charged on these overdrafts. If anybody thinks that Boris Johnson will have any concrete initiatives to invest in the future of the NHS, or in the wages of the nurses and doctors who saved his life, I think they will be disillusioned. And they deserve to be. The new normal will be austerity chapter 2 – or is it chapter 3? Austerity for the majority, of course, but more indulgence, more luxury, bigger yachts, and more whoopee parties for the great and the good that manage these things for us all.

Notes

1 Rajeev Jayaswal and Anisha Dutta, 'Centre rejects tax hike proposal by IRS officials, calls it ill-conceived', *Hindustan* Times, 26 April 2020, www.hindustantimes.com/india-news/centre-dismisses-tax-super-rich-proposal-by-irs-officials-calls-it-irresponsible/story-lJ6haLkNydtIzMNcm7gXNI.html (accessed 1 June 2020).
2 'CBDT initiates inquiry on IRS officers for unsolicited report on funding COVID relief work', *Economic Times*, 26 April 2020, https://economictimes.indiatimes.com/news/economy/policy/cbdt-initiates-inquiry-on-irs-officers-for-unsolicited-report-on-funding-covid-relief-work/articleshow/75393881.cms?from=mdr (accessed 1 June 2020).
3 *FORCE 1.0 (Fiscal Options & Response to COVID-19 Epidemic): Recommendations of the Indian Revenue Service on revenue mobilization and economic impetus to fight COVID-19* [unofficial IRS report]. 2020.
4 A couple of weeks after this was written, Prime Minister Narendra Modi announced a Rs.200 Lakh Crore Covid-19 relief package, around 10% of GDP, 'India fights Covid-19: PM Modi announces Rs 20 Lakh Cr Atmanirbhar Bharat package', *Economic Times*, 12 May 2020, https://economictimes.indiatimes.com/news/politics-and-nation/india-fights-covid-19-pm-modi-announces-rs-20-lakh-cr-atmanirbhar-bharat-abhiyan-package/videoshow/75701461.cms (accessed 2 June 2020). The kind of measures it was put to – with a strong emphasis on giving credit – bore no resemblance to what the unofficial IRS report had proposed.
5 Anthony B. Atkinson, *Inequality: What Can Be Done?* (Cambridge MA: Harvard University Press, 2012); Paul Krugman, *End This Depression Now!* (New York: W.W. Norton, 2012); Thomas Piketty, *Capital in the Twenty-First Century*, trans. Arthur Goldhammer, (Cambridge, MA: Harvard University Press, 2014 [2013]); Joseph Stiglitz, *The Price of Inequality* (New York: W.W. Norton, 2012).
6 Vivek Agnohotri dir., *Buddha in a Traffic Jam*, 2016, www.imdb.com/title/tt1890363/; Vivek Agnihotri, *Urban Naxals* (Gurugram: Garuda, 2018).
7 Tom Wheelwright, '5 ways that billionaire Warren Buffett pays a lower tax rate than his secretary', *Entrepreneur*, 30 August 2020, www.entrepreneur.com/article/338189.
8 Iain Duncan Smith, 'Iain Duncan Smith: Here's to a quiet success in the struggle against the virus – the resilience and robustness of universal credit', *Conservative Home*, 23 April 2020, www.conservativehome.com/platform/2020/04/iain-duncan-smith-why-universal-credit-is-working-better-than-ever.html. Smith was Secretary of State for Works and Pensions, 2010–2016, and oversaw the implementation of the centralized Universal Credit system replacing the prior benefits system. It had the effect of reducing the benefits of numerous claimants, making claims difficult to make and process, and other problems which have been prolifically reported in the news. It continued to be a problem over the Covid-19 lockdown period; see: Miles Brignall, 'Universal credit: "Almost impossible" to complete claim as more than 500,000 apply', *Guardian*, 26 March 2020, www.theguardian.com/world/2020/mar/26/universal-credit-claims-almost-impossible-as-more-than-500000-apply; Anoosh Chaklian, 'New to claiming universal credit? Here are its worst flaws', *New Statesman*, 27 March 2020, www.newstatesman.com/politics/welfare/2020/03/claiming-universal-credit-how-system-payments-delay (accessed 2 June 2020).
9 Johns Hopkins, 'University of Medicine, coronavirus resource centre', https://coronavirus.jhu.edu/map.html (accessed 2 June 2020).
10 'Triage', *Wikipedia*, https://en.wikipedia.org/wiki/Triage (accessed 2 June 2020).

11 Michel Foucault, *The Birth of Biopolitics: Lectures at the Collège de France, 1978–1979* (Basingstoke: Palgrave Macmillan, 2008).

12 'Arvind Kejriwal gives list of what's allowed in Delhi in lockdown 3.0' (video), *NDTV*, 3 May 2020, www.youtube.com/watch?v=N5RPEJQ9y8k (accessed 2 June 2020).

13 'Assessor de Eduardo Bolsonaro criou página do 'gabinete do ódio', diz site', *Poder360*, 4 March 2020, www.poder360.com.br/congresso/assessor-de-eduardo-bolsonaro-criou-pagina-do-gabinete-do-odio-diz-site/ (accessed 1 May 2020).

14 Terrence McCoy, Marina Lopes and Teo Armus, "This will not stick': Brazilian president lashes out over alleged links to left-wing politician's killing', *Washington Post*, 30 October 2019, www.washingtonpost.com/nation/2019/10/30/jair-bolsonaro-marielle-franco-murder-link/; Tom Phillips, 'Bolsonaro attacks "putrid" media over Marielle Franco murder claims', *Guardian*, 30 October 2019, www.theguardian.com/world/2019/oct/30/brazil-jair-bolsonaro-marielle-franco-murder-suspects (accessed 1 May 2020).

15 'Vídeo: Roberto Jefferson defende guerra civil para manter Bolsonaro', *Forum*, 29 April 2020, https://revistaforum.com.br/noticias/video-roberto-jefferson-defende-guerra-civil-para-manter-bolsonaro/ (accessed 2 June 2020).

INDEX

For Product Safety Concerns and Information please contact our EU
representative GPSR@taylorandfrancis.com
Taylor & Francis Verlag GmbH, Kaufingerstraße 24, 80331 München, Germany